FOOD
POWER

This book is dedicated to
Christine
for her
courage and great heart

With gratitude to Deva and Kashi, Brendon and Lyn
for their support
on many levels, material and spiritual.

FOOD POWER

Abhita & Iskaan

Zenzing Mystery School &
Gold Coast Natural Therapies

email:

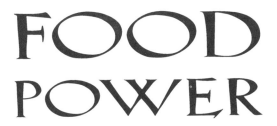

Healthybitz
Magnetic Therapy Products
Banwell House, Old Fore St.
Sidmouth EX10 8LP
Tel: 01395 578150
Email: healthybitz@supanet.com

The Oracle Press

Published by The Oracle Press
P.O. Box 121 Montville Qld 4560 Australia

National Library of Australia

ISBN 1 876494 06 9

Previous Publications

Beyond Degeneration, 1990
The Zinc Link, 1991
Astrobiochemistry - Towards Regeneration, 1994

Printed by Watson Ferguson & Co., Moorooka, Qld. 4105

CONTENTS

—◆— FOREWORD —◆—

Body Consciousness is a comprehensive physical and esoteric science which encompasses many modalities. In this book we are offering practical information concerning digestion and absorption of food together with many pages of wonderful recipes produced by Iskaan, both in our own kitchens and at healthy food demonstrations, in a frenzy of creative succulence.

Abhita's work is based on her own experience and observation of the many thousands of people that she has worked with. She has personally rid herself of arthritis and cancer and, diagnosed infertile, became a mother at 39. Her search started 22 years ago when, at the age of 30, she was severely crippled with arthritis. She was on heavy drugs and unable to move without pain.

Abhita read a book on juice fasting and tried it out. Within 10 days she could walk for the first time in two years. She was determined to find out what had gone wrong with her body and why nothing else had been able to help. She started to study Naturopathy, and as she learnt she experimented on herself.

Within a year the arthritis was gone, but her weight had risen to 119 kg. Using her own unique urindiagnosis method to present a picture of her body's functioning she discovered that her body was having great difficulty producing pancreatic digestive enzymes. When she started to balance this by taking appropriate enzyme supplements and separating out the heavier types of food, the excess weight began to drop off.

Abhita has streamlined her urindiagnosis test based on 15 years of empirical observation in her clinics and sessions all over the world.

She is the author of three books: *Beyond Degeneration*, *The Zinc Link*, and *Astrobiochemistry - Towards Regeneration*.

Iskaan is a biochemist and teacher whose study into the dietary requirements for optimum health was based on the observations of the functioning of his own body and those of his pupils while living on a 'normal' Western diet.

The resulting emotional and spiritual imbalance and lack of energy gave rise to a desire to find the way to access spirit-body harmony. His own search into the spirit-body link led to the union with Abhita and to working with Body Consciousness which satisfied both the scientific and esoteric aspects of his search. In the process he has cleansed and repaired his own body from the accumulated wastes and damage to the organs from diet, smoking and stress.

Chapter 1

DIGESTIVE ENZYMES

There are many thousands of enzymes in our bodies and in the foods that we eat, however, they all do different and specific jobs. The only enzymes which initially digest starches and fatty acids (after the ptyalin in our saliva has done its work) are pancreatic enzymes.

Namely, protease, lipase and amylase. These are not made anywhere else but in the pancreas except for the occurrence in small quantities in the small intestines and in mushrooms.

This book is written for people who do not make enough of these enzymes to match the kind of food they are eating and the lifestyle which they are trying to enjoy.

After testing many thousands of people and always finding a pancreatic enzyme deficiency we decided it would be interesting to research why this is so. Three main factors presented themselves over and over again, namely, environment, fear and of course, the food we have available in these times.

It is our information that we are responsible for everything that happens in our lives, we cannot put the burden of recovery onto anyone else's shoulders. If we acknowledge this, we may also understand that we have allowed ourselves to have a digestive enzyme deficiency for a reason.

It seems to us that the main reason we have done this is in order to lift our bodily vibrations to a state where we will be able to listen more easily to the spiritual information which is readily available to all of us.

This information has a very high vibration and if we put low vibrational foods into our systems, such as dead meat, chemicals, highly acid-forming foods and tobacco, our own body vibrations take these on too. We are then unable to listen to our higher selves, that is, our intuition, and we lose our way. We forget what we have come here to do, and we start to live lives of quiet desperation. Knowing vaguely in the back of our minds that there is something better somewhere, but not seeming to be able to access the information to act upon it.

Cleansing our systems, and putting natural mineral mixtures in to re-balance ourselves is the best way to start accessing this higher information which we all have. Then we can start to become the beings which we were created to be and live in harmony with others and with our surroundings.

We seem to choose places to live in which are not geographically suitable for human bodies. We do not generally live in love and honesty and an absence of these always creates fear and we do not generally eat real food.

Originally we were intended to live in temperate zones where the weather is warm enough for people to wander around without clothes and not feel cold. This enables a feeling of connection to all the things that surround us, feeling the sun on our skins, feeling the salty water of the seas, feeling the grass beneath our feet, feeling the breeze in our hair.

This all gave us a feeling of harmony and oneness with the other living parts of our surroundings and in this case we would never have presumed to set out to destroy or interfere with any of the other living things around us. Nor would we have poured into our environment the kind of pollution that we have if we could still feel really in touch with it. Because of our separation from our surroundings, however you choose to believe it came about, we learnt a new thing called fear.

Fear developed first through fear of losing the people we considered belonged to us, then through fear of losing what we considered to be our possessions, then through fear of losing what we considered to be our territory and so it went on. Actually fear is the absence of love and trust and brings with it all the other negative things like lust for greed and power, etc.

In recent times, since the first world war, fear has been universal and the media have made sure that never a day goes by without perpetuating it by bringing in living colour into our homes all kinds of events from all over the world which are guaranteed to cause fear.

The pancreas, the kidneys and the lungs are the seat of fear in our bodies and so they have constantly responded to this onslaught by lessening their efficiency. Since the First World War the pancreatic deficiencies, asthma and breathing difficulties and many kydney problems have been more and more noticeable.

Mustard gas, which was also used for the first time during that war, particularly affects that part of the pancreas which produces enzymes and the linings of the lungs and kidney tubules. This then becomes an inherited problem, which gets progressively worse as it is handed down from generation to generation without any repair work being done.

People migrate from the warm temperate zones to live in places that are either too hot or too cold and so they use clothes to protect them from these extremes. This negates straight away one of the main elimination processes, e.g., the huge area of the skin.

The skin still continues to eliminate but the clothes do not allow natural cleansing and evaporation of the toxins, so they and the acid, which comes out with them, dry on the skin. When the person heats up the acid also heats up and starts to burn. The person may get very itchy and wonder what they are allergic to. It's not an allergy; it's merely a condition of the way we live now. Because we tend to live in places that are either too hot or too cold or too dry or too wet our bodies have to try and compensate by asking for food other than that which was intended for it, namely cooked or frozen.

Our bodies were intended to process fruit and vegetables raw and possibly nuts and seeds. These were grown in abundance in an unpolluted atmosphere in a non-chemical world.

The pancreas was never intended to produce enough enzymes to digest the huge complex meals which we shovel into our bodies, let alone the fact that these foods are usually full of chemicals and cooked in hot fat or frozen solid.

It was intended to produce enough enzymes to digest a small amount of some kind of food at a time. If we eat like this every 2 or 3 hours then we do not have any enzyme problems. If we eat any other way then we are in trouble. We do not have the bowels of meat-eaters, which are short and straight as in dogs. We have long, undulating bowels, with very stretchy and permeable sides, these are the bowels of the plant-eaters and if we wish to return to good health that is just what we mainly have to be.

When we eat and drink things which our body can't process those substances stay in the body, fermenting, causing toxic matter to be retained in the body cells keeping those cells in darkness - depriving them of vital nutrients and oxygen.

To return to optimum health we have to address the other two main problems. That is, we must live where our bodies are comfortable. In that way we are not using all our energy just to keep warm or cool and to digest totally unsuitable food. Also we have to look at the fear in our lives and make determined efforts to eradicate it.

If, through eating and drinking food which our body can use to cleanse, nourish and energize our entire being, we can begin to access the fact that we are love, then we can stop looking for it outside of ourselves.

Chapter 2

DEGENERATION

The physical beginning of a degenerative disease is the poor absorption of food. Even if a perfectly balanced meal is eaten, if the body cannot break it down and absorb, it that person can be suffering from malnutrition. If the food cannot be broken down sufficiently to be processed into useable body components, then we have to ask ourselves what is happening to it? If the body cannot use it where does it go?

So you think it may all be excreted through the bowels, the skin and the kidneys - wrong! Much of it stays in the system and invades many of the healthy cells, eventually causing degeneration and disease.

The fully processed rubbish from just three normal-sized meals with all their complex mixtures would mean emptying the bowels about five times daily.

If digestive juices and enzymes do not break down the food, it will start to ferment. This fermentation produces a lot of bubbles and a lot of acid. The bubbles may be experienced as wind or burping, or both, as grumbling around the small intestines or as bloating around the stomach or bowel areas. This degeneration or fermentation of the undigested food is taking place at the top of the small intestines.

The acid from the fermenting food may be sent upward through the stomach, bronchioles and other mucous passages or downward throughout the entire small and large bowel system. This system of mucus-covered linings is actually connected from the nose to the anus with many side branches along the way.

When the acid from the undigested food hits the mucous lining it throws out mucus to protect itself. So we get mucus pouring into the system, especially above the stomach where the body has tried to force the acid back up to the oesophagus and out of the system.

This can result in many problems:

Hiatus hernia. As the acid burns the lining on the way back up the system over and over again, thinning it out and eventually allowing complete cell deterioration.

Bronchial congestion or even asthma. As the acid from the undigested food causes more and more mucus to be formed, it is forced back into the bronchials and even into the bronchioles to get it all out of the way. It then only requires a sudden shock such as the intake of cold air or an emotional crisis to constrict the tubes even further so that there is then no more room for air to pass through. Wheezing, coughing, choking and even asphyxiation may occur.

Allergies or allergic reactions. We do not generally agree that we are allergic to the actual substance consumed. We find that the symptoms may be alleviated with homoeopathic remedies but that the cause still needs to be investigated.

When a substance is put into the body and not digested, one of the things that happens is that some of it is absorbed into the blood stream. This is then present in different chemical formation than it would have been had it been digested properly. The allergic reaction then sets in as the body tries to rid itself of the apparent intruder as it does not have any instructions for this set of chemical patterns. The allergic reaction can take almost any form from mild to extremely severe.

An ingested substance causing an allergic reaction may cause nausea, vomiting, stomach cramps, severe wind or burping, dizziness, blurred vision, muddled thinking, severe mood swings, and fits, etc. These are all reactions which also occur as the results of undigested starches and fatty acids when there is a lack of digestive enzymes from the pancreas.

Fungal type reactions also occur when there are undigested starch and fatty acids in the mucous lining of the intestines where these types of organisms are generally found.

We have found that *candida albicans* is only completely eradicated when juice cleansing and following of the food list and separation of the heavy foods are undertaken. Also supplements must be taken, notably digestive enzymes, slippery elm, etc. The symptoms may be relieved quite fast with the homoeopathic remedies, but will probably eventually recur unless the other steps are taken.

Herpes and cold sores. This is one more problem we should like to give special mention. We have found quick relief from this condition occurs when the food of the person is changed and complete digestion ensured.

Herpes is a problem that occurs when zinc is deficient in the system. The sores usually appear when the person is under some kind of stress or pressure. Stress uses up huge amounts of zinc and other minerals. When the zinc is not being absorbed out of the food because it is not being digested sufficiently to allow it to be extracted, the protein absorption is also impaired.

An amino acid called L-Lysine is then also not absorbed properly. When supplements of both zinc and L-Lysine are given, with a properly separated and digested diet, the condition can improve overnight.

There are also herbs such as *Solanum Nigrum* as an ointment which help with this condition to relieve the discomfort when applied topically. We would encourage each of you to find a natural therapist who will work with enzyme and mineral therapy. Every single person is unique and so every single person's problems and method of treatment are going to be slightly different.

Hay fever. When the mucous linings are constantly aggravated by acids from undigested food, the inhalation of another foreign and irritating substance is enough to set off an immediate further mucus response. Together with other symptoms, sneezing, coughing, streaming nose and running eyes the body tries to rid itself as quickly as possible of the invading substance.

Middle ear infections. The mucus caused by the acid from the undigested fermenting foods backs up as far as the eustachian tubes, together with cholesterol (wax) from unprocessed fatty acids. The anaerobic germs and viruses then arrive in vast numbers and set up home for as long as this outpouring of mucus persists. This is why middle ear infections are particularly insistent.

If the mucus is still being produced, even after conventional medical treatment, a new set of bacteria will soon arrive to take the place of the previously evicted ones. Ear candling is a wonderful relief for this problem.

Sinusitis. This occurs when the mucus is backed up through the sinus cavities, causing pressure on and inflammation of the many nerves which run through those areas. These nerves can affect teeth, gums, ears and eyes and cause severe headaches and depression.

If the food is not broken down sufficiently, it cannot be further processed into the many chemical compounds which are needed for every single body function. Every part of the body is made up of the chemically broken down mineral mixtures from our food, our vital organs, our bones, our skin, our blood and especially our hormones.

If these mixtures go out of balance because the mineral components cannot be extracted from the food then any part of our body, which is already in a weakened condition because of inherited faults, is going to become worse. If the hormones are not fed the correct mineral mixtures they very quickly go out of balance. This means that all the messages they are supposed to send all over the body are also going to be out of balance, causing even more chemical disorders.

Some of the results of this are:

Menstrual disturbances. The zinc-copper ratio in the female body is very finely balanced. If not enough zinc is being absorbed from the food because it is not being broken down sufficiently, then this ratio is going to go out of balance. This is the main cause of premenstrual disturbances. If the zinc levels are already low, which they are in most of us, strange, depressive or even manic behaviour may result.

Infertility. This can be caused in many cases by poor absorption of minerals, especially zinc, leading to an imbalance in the reproductive systems causing difficulties in fertilisation and implantation.

If we finally get the egg fertilised and it embeds in the wall of the uterus, the cells start to divide very rapidly as the foetus forms. The very first thing that develops therefore must be a means to absorb nutrients into this new cell-cluster.

The first organs to develop are the pancreas and the salivary glands. At first they are joined together and as the foetus matures and becomes more complex, they become separate and assume separate functions.

So our very first inherited function is how many digestive

enzymes the pancreas is going to produce per stimulus of ingested food.

This is a genetically inherited function and cannot be changed.

—◆—— Chapter 3 ——◆—

BASIC DIGESTIVE
PROCESSES

W e put the food into our mouths and go chomp, chomp, swallow. The food lands in our top stomach and if we're lucky a hydrochloric acid solution is secreted through the stomach lining and starts to break down the proteins.

An intrinsic factor is released and absorption of B12 and other protein components starts to take place. What happens to the rest of the food? Well, nothing else is actually broken down for absorption in the stomach. All the other food is mulched up and passes down past the pancreas to the top of the small intestines where it is supposed to be showered with digestive enzymes from the pancreas. Now, if our genetically inherited quota of these enzymes is deficient for the amount of starches and fatty acids, which we are ingesting, then we're in trouble right from the start. Remember, there's nothing we can do to change the amount of these enzymes that we release as the food passes, so the only alternative we have is to change the food to suit our enzyme quota.

How can we tell whether we're making enough pancreatic enzymes to suit our intake of starches (sugars, carbohydrates) and fatty acids?

If the food is not broken down within a certain space of time, fermentation is going to occur. This is going to cause bubbles (a lot). This will manifest in wind or burping (colic in babies). If the wind is smelly then the proteins are also not digesting properly or else too much protein is being taken per meal. The fermentation of the undigested starches and fatty acids also causes a great deal of acid. This acid may go up or down the digestive tract, burning the mucous lining and causing it to throw out lots of mucus to protect itself.

Our next symptom is going to come from the gall bladder. The fatty acids should travel from the top of the small intestines after they have been broken down, to the gall bladder where the bile breaks them down even further into useable components which are then sent elsewhere.

However, if the fatty acids are not broken down in the first place, they will arrive at the gall bladder still raw and they will start to burn the cells of the gall bladder. This in turn clumps the offending substances together and surrounds them with a cholesterol mixture which stops their harmful effects. They are then stored around the gall bladder area or even in it, if they are too large to send back with the fatty acids which have been processed. If this happens often enough, gravel and stones will be formed in the gall bladder causing a whole new set of problems.

Although the gall bladder is only a tiny organ, when it becomes inflamed or aggravated in any way it can have many and various effects all over the body. It can be a kind of pain-referral centre, depending on where the gravel or stones are putting pressure, or which internal gall bladder cells are actually inflamed.

Symptoms of gall bladder aggravation may be as diverse as a very sharp pain in either big-toe, a sharp pain on breathing, so that the person is afraid to take a deep breath (sometimes mistaken for a heart attack), sharp pains under or between the shoulder blades (particularly the right-hand one). Other symptoms are pins and needles in hands or arms, bad pre-menstrual symptoms, restless legs (especially at night when trying to sleep), getting up around 3 o'clock in the morning to go to the toilet, tight shoulders and neck, migraine or cluster headaches, especially over the right eye, nausea and bloating, lack of appetite in the morning, tiredness on waking, lots of dreams and nightmares, short temper, a lot of wind, diarrhoea or constipation, very light-coloured stools which float, difficulty in digesting eggs and bananas.

None of these symptoms may mean that there is anything wrong with the gall bladder itself but they will mean that there have been raw fatty acids presented to this organ. So you would have to ask yourself why this is so, and the next thing to look at would be the pancreatic enzyme production and leaky gut syndrome.

As we stated before, these enzymes process starches and fatty acids, and if the fatty acids are not sufficiently broken down at this first stage they will arrive at the gall bladder raw and aggravate it, causing some or all of the above reactions. This is not initially a gall bladder problem; it is an enzyme problem!

The next symptoms of pancreatic enzyme deficiency we should look at are the results of the liver being overworked and undernourished. This happens because if the food is not sufficiently broken down to be used properly, the liver is then trying to do all the hundreds of different jobs it does, being involved in practically every function of the body, without the correct input of raw materials. This also adds to the poor functioning of the gall bladder, as the liver is too tired and does not have sufficient raw materials to make a good quality bile to send through to the gall bladder to aid in the breakdown and absorption of the fats.

The first message the body gives us that the liver is not being sufficiently nourished is *tiredness*, especially first thing in the morning. If this is ignored over a period of time, we become prime candidates for glandular fever and eventually chronic fatigue syndrome. After the tiredness has been ignored, the headaches will start. If these are ignored long enough, sleeplessness will set in, bringing with it a whole new set of problems. The reason that all these start to occur is that if the food is not being digested initially by the pancreatic enzymes, the liver will then try to take responsibility for breaking it down to a level where it can obtain useable material from it. This means that instead of stopping work at 2 a.m. it is struggling on until about 5 a.m. The person then falls into their deep sleep just before most of us have to get up, and consequently when they are roused, they feel really tired because, in effect, they have only just gone to sleep. The dreams and nightmares are readily remembered because when the liver is working, we are not able to go into our deep unconscious sleep.

The next organ we would have to look at to determine pancreatic enzyme deficiency is the thyroid gland. The liver and the thyroid gland reflect each other, that is, the way one functions offsets the way the other one functions. So the first symptom here is going to be the same as the first symptom for the liver and that is *tiredness.*

Here we have to look at exactly the opposite symptom also and that is *over-activity.* This is not just when a person seems to achieve an awful lot of things in a short space of time; rather, this over-activity is frenetic, disordered and out of control, very often not achieving much at all. The person feels driven on in spite of themselves.

The connection between this imbalance in the thyroid activity and pancreatic enzyme production is as follows: If the food is not broken down sufficiently, then the mineral mixtures are not able to be absorbed into the system. Hormones are made out of mineral mixtures. If the minerals are not absorbed in a balanced way then the hormone mixtures are going to be unbalanced.

The thyroid in particular relies on precise mixtures of minerals in the two main hormones it is concerned with, thyroidinum and thyroxinum. If these are not balanced within themselves and with each other then all the messages and jobs, which the thyroid is involved with, are going to go *out of balance*. Again, this does not mean that there is anything basically wrong with the thyroid gland itself, it just means that it is not being fed properly and therefore cannot function properly.

Another very early symptom that something is amiss with the liver, gall bladder or thyroid gland is *headaches*. Headaches solely on the right side or over the right eye or in a cluster over the right side of the head are usually associated with the gall bladder being aggravated. This, of course, is going to be associated with non-absorption of an intake of fatty acids, which is a pancreatic enzyme deficiency symptom, as the two main food groups which they are supposed to break down are starches and fatty acids.

The other food which has been shown to aggravate the liver, gall bladder and thyroid as well as the adrenals is **caffeine**. When you have a liver symptom in the morning such as tiredness or crankiness and you feel better after a cup of coffee, this is telling you how really undernourished this part of your system is. It needs to be artificially stimulated with such a heavy drug before you can begin to function properly. Caffeine is present in large quantities in many commonly used substances apart from straight coffee. Chocolate being the next most common form closely followed by tea and Coca Cola.

If you take any of these substances every day and feel better afterwards then you can be reasonably sure that your liver is tired, your minerals are out of balance, and so is your *blood-sugar*. Your body tends to crave these stimulants when your blood-sugar is low. It is actually trying to give the message that you need some minerals, but we translate that in our minds to needing a quick pick-me-up, so we have a caffeine or a sugar hit or both.

These are all symptoms of digestive enzyme deficiency, if we are digesting all our food, there should be enough minerals and slowly releasing sugars in our system to cope without needing these quick doses of artificial stimulants. This brings us to our next symptom: hypoglycaemia.

If we are absorbing all our food then the sugars release slowly into our bloodstream and keep a balance between our intake and our usage of sugars. If we are deficient in pancreatic enzymes which break down the starches and fatty acids, then the starches from which we obtain the sugars are not going to be broken down and our bodies will keep asking for more. Although we might have put them into our systems, they can not be used if they are not broken down and the body will then request more. It gives us this message by hitting a low as we run out of useable blood-sugars, so we get cranky, irritable, get blurred vision, confused or even blackout.

Age-onset diabetes is very closely related to this symptom as it is merely a pancreatic enzyme deficiency, which has been ignored or untraced over the years. This has led to the gradual weakening of the pancreas as the food, which it finds hard to cope with, is constantly being put in. This puts stress on the other function of the organ, which is to produce insulin. After many years of this happening, day after day, the pancreas becomes tired and undernourished and the insulin production goes down hill.

Age-onset diabetes should never occur. A person is either born with diabetes or they are not. It is not a true disease, but rather a sign that the body is degenerating and something should be urgently done to fix it up.

Overweight and underweight. These are both often caused by pancreatic enzyme deficiencies. The other particular inherited factors of each person determining whether the undigested deteriorating foodstuff is stored on the outside of the body-frame or thrown straight out through the bowel system.

In overweight, the person is constantly hungry because the food they are eating in response to brain signals from the appestat centre is not being digested, not being absorbed and so the body is constantly undernourished and will keep on asking for more nutrition with which to work.

There are quite a few ways in which the body deals with the undigested food to cause an overweight condition. In some people the undigested fermenting food is so undigested that it is recognisable in the faeces, i.e., sweet corn, peas, peanuts and raisins; all very heavy starch foods. In these kind of people what often happens is that because the food is not properly mulched up in the intestines the fluid that is available to assist in this mulching process cannot be used and so is reabsorbed along with fluid from the faeces themselves through the bowel lining. This is a very permeable membrane and is actually meant to be absorbing minerals and other nutrients from the final stages of digestion in the small intestines. This fluid is then absorbed into the intra-cellular fluid making the gaps between the cells larger and larger, with the person then looking bigger and bigger. In this case there may not be huge amounts of fat on this person, but huge amounts of *fluid*.

When the problem is recognised and proper food separation and a cleansing programme worked out, this excess weight will come off very fast and many toxins will be brought out with the fluid.

This fluid-type weight problem sets up another difficulty in that while moving the cells further away from each other they are also moved further away from the bloodstream and its life-giving nutrients. So while the person may look enormous and appear to be eating every five minutes, they are actually suffering from *malnutrition* and *exhaustion* as they are carrying around this enormous quantity of fluid which is very heavy. They are not receiving enough nutrition for themselves, let alone to do this great task of constantly carrying heavy weights.

This also causes many *skeleto-muscular* problems, as in standing, sitting and lying down, the fluid is constantly pulling the muscles into places where they were not designed to be and putting pressure on places which were not designed to take pressure. This means that person can never truly rest as their muscles are always in tension in response to the weight.

This removal of the fluid from the faeces also means that the material, which is left in the bowels, is very dry and consequently very hard to move by the peristaltic action of the bowels alone and this will form the hardest type of constipation. This holds the toxins formed by the decaying matter in the bowels for a long time and allows a lot of them to be re-absorbed through the bowel lining instead of the urgently needed minerals.

So these people are almost certain to have headaches, dizziness, lack of concentration, forget acquired knowledge like people's names and telephone numbers, also many have spatial difficulties, like knocking into things or sense difficulties like dropping things or misjudging distances. Many will also find their eyesight getting more blurred as the condition goes untreated or mistreated by short sighted (also) physicians who will tell them to use their willpower and eat less, possibly giving them a high-protein diet.

Overweight can also be caused by an excessive consumption of *protein* if it is in excess of that person's requirements, i.e., a fairly sedentary person, one who does light physical work. Unless we are lumberjacks or engaged in other such heavy physical endeavours we need only very small amounts of protein and that should be of any easily digestible nature such as mushrooms, broccoli, cauliflower, tofu or other fermented soy products. Harder to digest foods such as nuts, eggs, fish, etc., but certainly rarely red meat or full cream dairy products which most systems find totally indigestible and will store on the body as *fat.*

This type of body-fat is the hardest to get rid of and must be painstakingly exercised off by regular and prolonged physical exercise. This type of excess from undigested animal foods also causes fluid problems in the lower half of the body as the kidney function is interfered with.

Overweight can also be caused by the starches and fatty acids not digesting and being stored straight into the body cells, this is also a direct result of a deficiency of digestive enzymes from the pancreas and this results in fatty deposits anywhere on the body. This type of person will generally have all the aggravated gall bladder symptoms also.

This type of retention in the body of undigested foodstuffs is likely to cause congestion of the lymph glands and blockage of or enlarged lymph nodes. This can become a dangerous situation as the lymph system transports away all the larger rubbish and when it gets clogged up that rubbish again has nowhere to go. Other places in the body will be found to deposit it, which are not necessary for the person's survival, such as the ovaries, (causing ovarian cysts) the uterus (causing fibroids) or around the joints, shoulders and neck (causing arthritic-type symptoms).

These lymphatic blockages attract other free radicals and toxic substances and may eventually become cancerous if not dealt with. The lymph system does not have a definite flow like most other systems of the body, but relies upon the pumping action of the diaphragm to send it around the body.

People who are overweight generally do not breathe very deeply as it is an extra effort to lift a diaphragm which is covered in heavy fat or fluid. Neither do they generally do a lot of aerobic exercise for the same reason. Because of this they may be more likely to end up with a cancerous situation in their bodies. All caused initially by an inherited lack of digestive enzymes - undiagnosed and untreated.

Underweight is caused when the undigested starches and fatty acids ferment, making even more acid. In these people the mucous linings are already so aggravated that the intestines peristalt rapidly to get rid of the offending substances, often sending a lot of mucus out with the faeces, as much will be generated along the way to protect the tender mucous lining from even further damage. These people consequently do not have time to absorb much of their food and so are also *constantly hungry* even though they may be described as 'eating like a horse and never putting on any weight'. They are also probably *mineral deficient*, as the food does not stay long enough in their bodies for them to absorb many of the minerals and nutrients through the small intestines.

These people may often suffer from *diarrhoea* as a consequence from losing a lot of fluid and becoming very thin. They may also have an itchy anus as the constant attack of acid coming out fairly raw will burn the anus as it passes through. This may also cause haemorrhoids as will the hard, dry constipated faeces of the fluidy, overweight person, due to the constant erosion of the lining by not only the dry faeces but also by the acids which cannot mix in with them. They come through fairly raw, burning the lining all the way, but especially around the anus where everything is concentrated.

Bladder infections, cystitis, bed-wetting. These are also caused initially by an enzyme deficiency from the pancreas. As the undigested food ferments and makes acid, much of this is sent out through the kidneys and urinary system. Because the acid is raw, the bladder will want to throw it out as soon as possible. In children, this is one of the main causes of bed-wetting. The bladder will not wait until it is full and then give the child the signal to wake up and go to the toilet. Instead, without any warning, it will just eject its contents as quickly as possible so that the irritation being set up may be avoided.

In adults, we may wake up before this occurs, but it means constant visits to the toilet throughout the night.

It is worse at night because little is being excreted through the skin compared to the amount we throw out in that way during the day. If the problem is severe, *itching of the legs* or *night sweats* may occur. All these should tell you that your kidneys are burdened with over-acidity from undigested foods. When this occurs constantly the mucus, which the body throws out to protect itself in this area may very quickly become infected, as it is all these undigested things in the mucus that the bacteria feed upon. This then turns from cystitis to a bladder infection.

In this area we also have to look at the problem of undigested protein. The proteins are broken down initially by a hydrochloric acid mixture in the stomach. This mixture is made partly in the pancreas and partly in the liver. If the pancreas function is already impaired and the liver is already overworked, then this mixture is not going to be sufficiently strong to digest heavy proteins.

After various other processes the prepared protein components reach the tiny tubules, which are involved with the kidneys. Here they are supposed to be absorbed through the linings into the bloodstream.

If these components are not broken down enough the particles will be too large and scrape the tubules on the way through, causing severe pain. If this situation is ignored the larger crystals (uric acid) from undigested meat and animal products, and other minerals which congregate in these areas, will clump together forming stones or gravel. The body may decide to deposit these crystals in the cavity areas of the joints - causing the pain and inflammation of arthritis and gout.

A common symptom of this is *stiffness* in the lower back in the morning. This is caused by the gravel collecting in one place as the person lies relatively still during the night, and when they try to move in the morning the crystals scrape the lining of the tubules hitting nerve endings and causing inflammation, pressure and pain. This is usually relieved after a hot shower and moving around as this breaks up the deposits and allows them to move on more freely. If this situation is ignored the stones or gravel may cause a complete blockage resulting in excruciating pain and a very dangerous condition.

Anywhere in the body where there is inflammation, large amounts of leucocytes are brought in to fight the problem including any infection which may be taking place. This depletes the body's energy and the immune system.

The immune system is made up largely of zinc together with other mineral components. If the enzymes haven't been breaking up the food sufficiently to get the mineral components which they need to make the correct mixtures for the immune system, then this most important function is not going to be able to operate properly.

The **adrenals**, which sit on top of the kidneys, also suffer where there is a lack of digestive enzymes. The adrenals use a hormone called adrenalin which is also made up of mineral components, and so for the same reasons given above, their many jobs cannot be performed properly without the right materials. When the adrenals suffer, we get *stressed out* very easily, lose our ability to react immediately in dangerous situations and women suffer badly during menopause.

Menopausal problems come about through three main deficiencies all traceable to a poor secretion of pancreatic enzymes. The three areas which are most important in this respect are the adrenals, the liver and the thyroid.

The liver is the main factory where the hormones are put together. The thyroid and the adrenals need the hormones with which to facilitate a smooth crossing over from ovulating to non-ovulating.

When the ovaries decide that they've produced enough eggs (all the eggs, by the way, are with us from birth, so it depends on what food we absorb as to what condition they are in when we ovulate) they send a message to the adrenals to take over the releasing of the oestrogen in a cyclic manner so that the body may remain stable and balanced.

The adrenals send a message to the liver that they will need more oestrogen and that the ovaries do not want any more. This message is also sent by a hormone as are all messages in the body (nerve cells receiving their messages across neuro-transmitter fluid which is made of hormones). So if the liver is too busy trying to do all the other things it has to do and not having the right mineral mixtures at the time, it will send back a *hot flush* as it tries to sort the whole thing out with not enough material.

The thyroid is involved because if its mineral mixtures are not correct it is not going to be able to play its part in the absorption of the calcium into the bones and osteoporosis will then occur. This can all be avoided and remedied by correcting the digestive and absorption problems. This brings us to the next part of the book, that of transition. This involves finding out what to do about everything and how to go about it and which bits to do first.

Chapter 4

WHAT TO DO

We need to remember that we are dealing with degenerative diseases, this is a drastic situation and requires urgent treatment. There are basically three approaches:

1. Juice cleansing for a couple of weeks and then continuing the cleansing on very light food.
2. Changing over of food. Separating the heavy foods out and avoiding many of the foods that were previously enjoyed.
3. Changing things slowly over a couple of years a little bit at a time.

It really depends what the problem is and how urgent it is to fix it up as to which way you decide to go. Obviously the first choice is the one which gives the deepest, quickest cleansing and will help change habits and attitudes much more easily. However, some people are not psychologically prepared for fasting and should not try to do anything like that until they are ready for it. Fasting is a skill in its own right and should never be undertaken on your own without experienced supervision. We do not agree with water fasting. In our opinion it depletes the body's energy reserves without giving anything back, releases all the toxins too dramatically, is quite painful and it takes some time to recuperate.

There are some people who do not agree with this point of view and so we shall agree to differ with them.

Juice cleansing on the other hand uses all the minerals from the plants, vegetables and fruits to supply the body with energy to do the cleansing and repair work all in one go. Instead of feeling utterly depleted at the end of the cleanse, the person is full of energy and ready to get on with their new life.

There are some very important rules to apply before you jump into a juice cleanse:

1. A cleansing, detoxifying fast requires complete rest and removal from the person's normal circumstances.
2. There should be absolutely no demands made on the person who is cleansing.
3. Emotional and spiritual counselling should be available to the person cleansing together with frequent use of Bach Flower Remedies to help break the old patterns and take away any negativity or fear which has come with the release of toxins from the body.

As the toxins are released and removed from the body, so are the old emotions and wounds which were involved in causing the state of disease in the first place. We invite disease into our bodies by being in a state of mind, which allows us to eat and drink foods which we know very well do not agree with us. Everything which happens to our bodies happens in our minds first.

When we are re-presented with these problems, which we ran away from the first time by pushing them down into our bodies, we need to have expert help available to surround these things with love. Have a good look at them and allow them to be healed.

The length of the cleanse depends on the previous life-style of the person, their mental attitude and their physical condition. The elimination is going to be very uncomfortable for the first few days, maybe even a week, if the person is starting their first ever cleansing and is used to drinking coffee, tea, alcohol, soft drinks, Coca-cola, cordials, etc., and eating red meat, fried or roast foods, sugar, white flour and white rice products. These people would need at least two weeks.

This would need to be followed up in a few months' time with another two-week juice programme and maybe even a third one a few months later depending on how everything was going.

There are many millions of cells in the body and every one of them is capable of holding toxic matter and of being interfered with by mineral imbalances. It takes a long time usually to realise and admit that something is radically wrong with our systems, and it usually takes a long time to put it completely right again, but it can be done.

The body is capable of fixing, regenerating and repairing just about any problem given the right materials and conditions to work with. This definitely includes an absence of stress, which is why it is so important to change our attitudes and habits along with our food and drink.

The need for complete rest during a juice cleanse is because the body uses an enormous amount of energy doing the cleansing. If we try to live on juice and carry on doing our normal activities we may lose a lot of weight and fluid, but we will not be cleansing; we will be starving.

The need for total absence of stress is because coping with stress uses up enormous amounts of minerals. When cleansing, these minerals are needed to provide energy and to do the repair work and cleansing, especially of the bowel area, and to feed the immune system, which sometimes has to work overtime during a deep cleansing.

If the person can handle it psychologically, a daily enema helps enormously to alleviate the discomfort brought about by the huge amounts of toxins being released into the system. An enema will facilitate removal of these toxins as soon as they are being released so that none get re-absorbed and cause headaches and arthritic aches and pains in the joints.

If a person is already underweight, the juices, which are normally taken three-hourly and diluted with pure water when necessary, are supplemented with liquid protein drinks. The composition of which depends on the condition of that person.

Meditation is encouraged. This facilitates the changing of habits and old learned attitudes which must go if the person is going to remain in good health once the cleanse is over.

Aromatherapy massage is a wonderful help during the cleanse, especially on the days when the person is not feeling too good or is releasing some heavy emotional stuff. The aromatherapy process is not only gently relaxing but assists the lymph to carry the toxins out of the little pockets that they've made for themselves. It also soothes all the nerves which can get aggravated during the deeper cleansing stages that occur every four or five days.

The oils sink into the body down the hair follicles over the areas where the problems are occurring and continue doing their healing cleansing work for up to a week depending on which mixtures have been used.

The second choice of finding out what is not digesting and changing the food to suit our quota of digestive enzymes with careful food separating becomes a life-time commitment to good health. This programme is what the juice-cleansers will go on to when they return home. Although no fasting is involved it is still a cleansing programme, and so at the beginning some discomfort may be noticed, again, depending on the previous life-style of the person.

Our urindiagnosis test shows in a matter of minutes the proportion of digestive enzymes to the amount of starches and fatty acids eaten. In other words, it tells how much of your food you are digesting. This test also shows the condition of the gall bladder and its function, the condition of the kidneys and their functions, the condition of the liver and many of its functions, the condition of the pancreas in general as well as specifically noting the state of the enzyme production, and the condition of the mucous linings throughout the body and of the bowels in particular. It can also show the condition of the male and female reproductive systems and their functions.

Of course, together with this test, many questions are asked and many other diagnostic methods used to get a whole picture of exactly why, how, and where the person is healthwise. There are many other methods of treatment also, depending on what the problem is, but we have found that whatever else is done the digestive enzyme deficiency has to be dealt with, by a change of food and careful separating of the heavy foods used. Otherwise the problem which the person has is only going to recur because the original cause, which is the poor absorption of the food, has not been addressed.

Depending on the degree of pancreatic enzyme deficiency and the condition of the body, an individual eating plan is made up especially for the person. However, we are including here a general eating plan which will benefit everybody, together with a plan of the way food can generally be separated.

Together with this, when a person first comes to be diagnosed there are generally herbal or other remedies and natural food supplements which they need depending on their problem. All supplements, mineral, vitamin or food, should always be as natural and as fresh as possible. There are many items sold in health food shops which have no right to be there.

Always consult your natural health practitioner about supplements as many are very expensive, quite unsuitable and may even be harmful if they are not natural.

FOOD LISTS AND GUIDELINES

A mixture of the following food sources every day in suitable combinations will easily supply our daily requirements. If repair work or extra cleansing is happening in the body, natural supplements may need to be taken for a short time.

Many minerals are water soluble, so if the food is steamed or boiled, the water will contain many of the minerals and can be consumed in a variety of ways so that the minerals are not lost.

MINERAL CHARTS

SOURCES OF IRON		
Livers	Prunes	Sesame seeds
Raspberries	Apricots (dry)	Black grapes
Molasses	Cherries	Red bush tea
Parsley	Beetroot	Eggs
Lentils	Pinenuts	Sunflower seeds
Almond kernels	Nectarines	Leafy greens - vegies
Peaches	Cashews	Red Clover & Alfalfa -
Figs (dried)	Plums	sprouts & Tea

CALCIUM	ZINC
Sesame seeds (whole)	Pollen granules
Parsley	Royal jelly
Almonds	Nuts
Figs (dried)	Seeds, especially
Watercress	pumpkin seeds
Eggs, calamari	Fish, shellfish
Broccoli (raw)	Poultry
Sunflower seeds	Livers
Cabbage	Eggs, mushrooms
Brussel sprouts	Yellow & green vegetables
Buckwheat	Yellow fruits - papaya,
Onions	mangoes
Hazelnuts	Sprouted seeds & nuts
Celery	Apples
Strawberries	Pears
Carrots	Carrots
Tofu	Lettuce
Lemons	

FOOD LIST	
AVOID	TRY
Red Meat	Chicken, turkey (free range, skin off), fish, game, eggs
Coffee, Tea, alcohol, Horlicks, Milo, Ovaltine, drinking Choc.	Herbal teas, lemon-grass, fennel, chamomile, mineral or soda water
White pastry, noodles	Wholemeal flour, bread or noodles
Wheat products	Corn, rye, millet
All forms of cane sugar	Honey
Processed cereal	Brown rice, rolled oats, millet
Processed meat	Nuts, seeds
Cheese	Soy cheese, tofu, low-fat fetta
Bacon, ham	Red lentils, tempeh (wheat free)
Oranges, orange juice	Other citrus fruits, pure juices
Chocolate	Unsweetened carob, dried fruit
Butter, margarine	Cold-pressed oils
White vinegar	Apple-cider vinegar
Artificial colouring, flavouring	Paprika, turmeric, tamari or miso, herbs & spices, pure vanilla
Preservatives	Lemon & lime juice, honey, vinegar
Salt, sauces	Spices, curry, tomato paste
Vegemite, Promite	Seasalt, hatcho miso (wheat-free)
(MSG) No. 621	Beansprouts, tahini, parsley, mint
Fried foods	Grilled, casseroled, steamed, roasted or baked (no oil) foods
Chips, lollies	Raw or steamed vegetables
Whole milk, cream	Sour light cream, soy milk
Ice cream	Fresh fruit, pureed frozen fruit
Cooked spinach, rhubarb	Leafy green vegetables
No heated oil or fat	Tamari (wheat-free), lemon juice

FOOD SEPARATING FOR EASIEST DIGESTION WHEN THERE IS A DIGESTIVE ENZYME DEFICIENCY

PROTEINS	*OR*	STARCHES
Only one at a meal		Only one at a meal
Buckwheat, beans, egg, fish, free range chicken & livers, free range turkey, olives, grains (brown rice, wild rice, millet) soybean products (miso, tofu, tempeh, wheat-free only), seeds, nuts, tahini (sesame seeds), rolled oats, sprouted and unyeasted bread, skim milk yoghurt, cereal.		Beans, buckwheat, carob, chestnuts, chick peas, couscous, coconut & coconut milk, grains (brown rice, wild rice, millet), lentils (red), parsnips, pasta, peas, potato, pumpkin, seeds, sweet corn, sweet potato, tapioca, nuts, rolled oats, yams, bread (unyeasted), cereal.

OR
FATTY ACID

Only one at a meal

Avocados, chicken and livers, coconut and coconut milk, eggs, fish, oils, olives, nuts, seeds, tahini and turkey.

Note
Only one type of protein or starch or fatty acid per meal with digestive enzymes.

FRESH VEGETABLES

Mix as you like with any Starch or Protein or Fatty Acid.

Asparagus	Bamboo shoots	Swede
Beetroot	Broccoli	Brussel sprouts
Cabbage	Herbs	Capsicum (red)
Red Onions	Zucchini	Radish
Carrots	Cauliflowers	Celery
Eschallot	Eggplant (ripe)	Snow-Peas
Garlic	Ginger	Green Beans
Spring onion	Okra	Kohlrabi
Leafy greens	Leeks	Squash
Turnips	Onions	Mushrooms
Watercress	Beansprouts	Tomato (egg)
Lebanese cucumber		

- Leave half an hour between fruit and vegetables.
- Never mix Fruit with Protein, Starch or Fatty Acid foods.

Acid Fruits	Sub Acid Fruits	Eat Alone
Grapefruit	Apricots, Apples (red, yellow)	Bananas
Limes	Blackcurrants, Blackberries	Custard apples
Mandarins	Cherries (sweet), Gooseberries,	Dried fruit
Pineapples	Grapes(small amount), Guava	Papaya
Sour plum	Loganberries, Loquats, Mangoes	Fresh figs
Lemons	Nectarines, Passionfruit, Peach	Melons
Tangerines	Pear, Pomegranate,	Dates
	Raspberries, Persimmons	Quinces
	Strawberries, Sweet plums	

• Do not mix these groups of fruits together.
• Avocados eaten on their own or with a green salad and enzymes.
• The 'Eat Alone' group should be eaten only one at a time and not mixed with anything else, followed by digestive enzyme tablets if required.

The following may be mixed with anything
• Lemons & limes, sour light cream, tamari sauce, apple cider vinegar, honey, pineapple, lo fat ricotta cheese, 100% fat-free skim milk.

The best way to use the food separation list is to work around the group of vegetables in the middle. These may all be mixed together, as much as you like, raw or cooked. However, together with these you may only use either one protein or one starch, or one fatty acid. Even if the starches are of vegetable origin, only one may be taken at a meal. If you still have any digestive enzyme deficiency symptoms as mentioned then you are a person who will need to take a pancreatic enzyme supplement.

---◆--- Chapter 6 ---◆---

FOOD VALUES AND PROBLEM FOODS

Whole or complete proteins are those that contain the eight amino acids which our bodies are mostly unable to synthesise so they must be obtained from our food. These amino acids are then used to make proteins, which are required by our bodies for specific tasks and if any are missing these functions will be impaired.

Mushrooms are a good source of whole proteins and Vit.B12, and are able to be digested without enzyme supplements, as they are the only one of the vegetables which contain the equivalent of pancreatic enzymes. They also may be mixed with anything though they do not contain the concentration of enzymes necessary to digest other proteins, starches or fatty acids.

Most vegetable proteins are considered nutritionally superior to animal proteins as they are more easily digested and therefore assimilated by the body. Sprouts are an excellent source of easily assimilated amino acids as the proteins have already been broken down ready for the plant's own growth needs.

Note that the benefits of any whole proteins are only available if the foods containing them are completely digested which makes the amino acids available. As digestive problems are due to a pancreatic enzyme deficiency, pancreatic enzyme supplements also containing betaine hydrochloride are essential for complete breakdown of the whole proteins, which are listed in the Food Separating Chart.

Nuts and Seeds

Nuts and seeds contain whole proteins, starch and fatty acids, making them a heavy combination, so only a few must be eaten at a time and not mixed with any other heavy food. They also contain an enzyme inhibitor which retards the digestion, so they must be lightly heated to inactivate the inhibitor. Heating should be done without oil (tamari may be used to stop sticking) and the nuts and seeds are then allowed to cool before eating.

Almonds are a wonderful source of calcium but the brown skin must be removed by blanching in hot water, as it contains large amounts of Tannin which eats away the stomach lining. This amount of heating is also enough to inactivate the enzyme inhibitor.

Peanuts contain aflatoxins which make them unsuitable for eating as they cause heavy allergic reactions, notably mucus streaming from the nose and middle ear infections. All nuts and seeds to be used in small quantities with digestive enzymes and not mixed with any other protein, starch or fatty acid.

De-chemicalising Vegetables and Fruit

It is always preferable to use organically grown produce wherever possible. If this is not available, several clear quartz crystals may be programmed to do the job of channelling out the chemicals. We have three in the fridge, some by the water and some in the fruit bowls. These need cleaning every week by soaking in seawater overnight and then being reprogrammed by connecting to the love within and telling them what is required.

Food List

You will notice that right at the top of the list is red meat. This is no accident. As mentioned before, we are not generally able to process red meat into useable components and it therefore becomes one of the biggest offenders in setting up and eventually causing degenerative disease.

We do not have the strength in the hydrochloric acid solution, which we secrete through the stomach lining, to break down red meat sufficiently. Dogs are able to digest red meat, their acid solution is many times stronger than ours is and their bowels are short and straight to eliminate the waste products.

So when we are putting red meat into our systems day after day rather, than reaping the benefits from a good whole protein, we are clogging up our systems as the meat starts to ferment and produces acid all the way through the digestive tract. It is slightly easier to absorb some of its nutrients when it is not cooked at all. As soon as it has been heated enough to cook it, the fatty acids contained in every fibre will change chemically to nitrosamines and these are capable of causing cancer in the bowel.

The fatty acids from animal products will also be a dietary source of arachidonic acid which will build up to produce many harmful and degenerative effects throughout the body including *hormonal* disturbances and *leaky gut syndrome*.

So straight away we are causing many problems, together with the fact that undigested red meat will also produce uric acid. This may settle around the joints if it cannot be excreted quickly enough, eventually causing inflammation because the uric acid crystals are very sharp. Every time the joint moves the crystals scrape nerve endings and arthritic inflammation and pressure set in, eventually causing much pain and stiffness.

Gout is related to this problem also, usually affecting the big toe first. This is a gall bladder symptom and happens because the stomach acids do not digest the meat in the first place, and the fatty acids are not digested in the second place because there is a lack of pancreatic enzymes which are supposed to digest starches and fatty acids.

Because of the fact that any heated fat or oil or butter changes chemically at certain temperatures, all fried food, foods roasted or baked in oil, must also be avoided, even if it is all vegetables! When people are first changing their food habits it is fine to include small amounts of cold-pressed oils as long as they are never heated.

Margarine and other vegetable oils have all gone through various chemical processes to extract, deodorise and make them an acceptable colour and smell and are quite unsuitable for inclusion in any diet.

Cholesterol is a naturally occurring sterol in the body, manufactured in the liver to assist in the transport of fats around the body. When we ingest a substance containing foreign cholesterol the whole balance is upset and the body tries to store the foreign cholesterol out of the way, usually around the arteries. Cholesterol is made in the liver and therefore can *only* be found in animal products. Fatty acids may be found in vegetables and nuts but never cholesterol.

The beginning of fatty acid digestion occurs with the pancreatic enzymes and if these are inadequate then we're in trouble right from the start.

On our list of 'avoids' the fatty acids mentioned are: red meat, processed meat, butter, cheese, bacon and ham, margarine and cooking oil, foods roasted or baked in oil, and fried foods, chips, whole milk and cream, icecream and heated oil or fat. This also includes any products which contain any of the above.

Cheese is a disaster to anyone with a deficiency of pancreatic enzymes. When it is undigested in the first place, it starts to ferment causing a lot of the *burning* kind of indigestion and the very uncomfortable kind of wind in the small and large intestines after it has been rejected by the gall bladder and sent back for excretion. There is a tendency for people changing from a meat-eating habit to become addicted to cheese instead. There is absolutely no advantage in this, as the cheese is setting up many of the same problems. An added problem with the cheese is the addition of the colourings and flavourings, some of which have been proved to be genetically damaging.

If people are looking at cheese or dairy products to give them calcium in their diets, then they should think again and go to foods which have readily assimilable calcium and are not going to do them any other harm. Skim milk yoghurt, low fat ricotta cheese, skim milk fetta and sour light cream are the only dairy sources of calcium which we include in our eating plan, and these are to be used sparingly. Raw broccoli and parsley, cabbage, sprouted almond kernels, watercress, etc., being good natural sources of calcium and many other minerals. Most nuts and seeds and many other vegetables and fruit contain calcium in varying amounts, so if we have a good mixture of raw fruits and vegetables every day, we can be sure of getting enough calcium for normal requirements.

If we do need extra calcium for any repair work or growth requirements to teeth and bones, etc., a supplement is available which is prepared with orotic acid. The orotic acid takes the already broken down calcium right through the digestive system and deposits it into the cells which need it the most urgently. This is particularly suitable for people who have digestive problems as all the digestive work has been done for them. This preparation is called Calcium Orotate (we also recommend Hydroxyapatite) and should come in a mixture with its co-factors which include D3, magnesium, manganese, iron, copper, zinc, B6, silica, ascorbic acid or betaine hydrochloride and kelp. It should, however, be used in conjunction with instructions from a qualified natural health practitioner.

Coffee and tea are next on the list. This is because these two products probably make up half or more of the person's average intake of liquid and both are totally destructive to the body's delicate balance and cause immeasurable damage to many of its functions. Caffeine is an addictive stimulant drug which can cause an overactive nervous system, can affect the heart rhythm, the diameter of the blood vessels, coronary circulation, blood-pressure and urination. It can encourage the adrenal system to overwork leading to chronic fatigue and can be involved in infertility. Removal of this drug from a person's diet will cause bad headaches; these will pass after about three days.

White flour, breads, cereals, pasta, pastry, noodles. These are all very congestive, energy-using products and should be completely avoided, especially for people who do not make enough pancreatic enzymes. Wholemeal rye, buckwheat, etc., may be alright to consume as flour, pastry, noodles or pasta. When the bran and other nutrients are removed, as they are in the white products, you are left with an empty starch, and this is just the very thing which is the hardest to digest. The bran, etc., contains the protein and B vitamins. When this is removed, in order for the rest of the product to be digested, it must take these, particularly the B vitamins, from the body's own stores.

So, not only are these white products highly indigestible to those with a pancreatic enzyme deficiency, but they are actually using the body's own supplies of B vitamins in order to process them. This is why they are so high up on the list of 'avoids'.

Also when they are not digested they start fermenting, making lots of acid and mucus and clogging up the bowels causing constipation and/or diarrhoea.

Grains are the means by which plants reproduce and grow

so they must contain all the necessary requirements for their growth, i.e., protein, starch and fats. All these nutrients together in one food are a heavy combination to begin with so they are difficult to digest without a large number of digestive enzymes. Grains should be eaten in small quantities, or preferably not eaten at all.

Bread. The grains are difficult to digest on their own but most bread contains more than one type of flour which is a heavy combination of different starches and proteins. Also thrown in is yeast, which we find most people have problems coping with, and sugar to help the fermentation process and oils. The resulting mixture is a very heavy combination which is completely indigestible. Alternatives which may work, are sprouted breads, buckwheat pan bread (buckwheat is a vegetable starch) or bread made from one type of grain only and no yeast or oil. These are best mixed only with salad or honey and taken with digestive enzymes.

Cane sugar and all its other refined names like glucose, dextrose, sucrose, etc., causes similar problems to white flour products. Again, we are left with an empty starch which depletes the body's own stores of B vitamins in order to even begin digesting it. But here we have an even more dangerous situation than the white flour products because the components of the cane sugar absorb into the bloodstream in large quantities not suitably broken down and interfere with the delicate messages for blood-sugar and insulin balance, causing hypoglycaemic, diabetic and other problems. As there is refined cane sugar in almost every manufactured edible product, this interference in our blood-sugar balance takes place almost every time we put anything manufactured into our mouths.

This causes wild mood swings, yawning and tiredness, dizziness and irrational behaviour. The tiredness in particular prompting the person to want to eat some more of the product to, hopefully, give them some more energy when in fact it is going to do exactly the opposite. This is even more of a problem when the person has a pancreatic enzyme deficiency as cane sugar is one of the heaviest starches and so is unable to be broken down for proper use in the system right from the start.

The best alternative to sugar is honey. This should preferably be raw and produced without heat and the addition of antibiotics. Although honey is a starch, it is not sucrose but levulose and is readily absorbed into the bloodstream without requiring such huge efforts of digestion. Real honey contains many natural enzymes and antibiotics which are very valuable. The components of honey also help to maintain and repair the myelin sheath around the nerves (which need as much help as they can get in these days of stress) and also give us instant useable energy.

Processed cereals are also denatured, heated and added to and are empty starches with little or no food value left in them. They require large amounts of digestive enzymes to cope with them, especially as they are usually taken with whole milk and cane sugar. People with a deficiency in these enzymes have absolutely no hope of digesting these type of foods. Rolled oats with honey followed by a digestive enzyme supplement is about the only alternative vaguely suitable, but only people living in a very cold climate or doing hard manual labour really need this type of food in the morning.

Mueslis are totally unacceptable as they are a mixture of so many proteins and starches that very little of the meal will be digested even if an enzyme tablet is taken. The original Swiss type muesli was a mixture of grated apple and grated nuts with honey and lemon juice, usually taken with biodynamic skim milk yoghurt. This is much more acceptable as the body's initial fuel for the day.

Chocolate contains a multitude of problems. Usually, it is

made with whole milk and cane sugar, together with vast numbers of artificial flavourings, colourings and preservatives, all compounding the original problem of the chocolate itself.

Chocolate contains caffeine and apart from causing all the problems that caffeine causes it also makes oxalic acid which attacks the linings in the large bowel and small intestines. This adds to the problem of leaky gut syndrome in the large bowel as do spinach and rhubarb when they are cooked. Raw spinach is alright in small quantities shredded into a mixed green salad or in small quantities in a mixed vegetable juice.

When a person craves for chocolate it is an immediate indication that their mineral levels are low (magnesium, zinc and tin in particular), and a large glass of carrot and celery juice taken straight away will usually take away the craving. The cause of the mineral deficiency should then be looked into. It will usually be traced to a digestive enzyme problem because if the food is not broken down properly the minerals from it are unable to be absorbed.

Another reason can be intestinal permeability, which means that we lose our nutrients through the bowel lining which has been damaged by acids from undigested foods, antibiotics and anti-inflammatory drugs. This will cause wind, bloating and tiredness as we are not able to use the nutrients in the form in which they are now circulating through our system. Instead, they will cause pockets of toxic matter to be formed and also clog up the circulatory systems causing a whole new set of malfunctions. Slippery Elm taken before food is of immeasurable help in these situations. Biodynamic skim milk yoghurt in small quantities may also be used to reintroduce the friendly bowel flora which keep our guts working smoothly.

When we are under stress our bodies use huge amounts of minerals to cope with it. If we are fighting off an infection of some kind at the same time or repairing some body damage which has been done, then the needed mineral input is very large. If we're not digesting our food, then those minerals are just not available. This problem is particularly noticeable in women between ovulation and menstruation when the mineral mixtures are needed and used in very large quantities and this is usually when the worst chocolate cravings set in.

Taking Royal Jelly at this time, together with a good, natural zinc and mineral mixture will help enormously to alleviate the cravings. If we don't supplement at these times when our bodies are obviously using more minerals than they are capable of absorbing out of the food, then our immune systems suffer and we tend to start catching whatever is currently going around.

Carob in its dry powdered form is 80 percent starch and a good source of calcium but being such a concentrated starch it must not be mixed with proteins, starches or fatty acids. Most carob products are mixed with milk, oils and fillers, making them impossible to digest, so these should be avoided. Read the ingredients and remember 'no added sugar' does not mean that the ingredients themselves do not contain sugar.

Oranges and orange juice are totally unsuitable especially for people who already have a mucus problem or an over-acid system because of undigested foods fermenting. Most acid foods, if digested, become alkaline and become very beneficial in the system, but oranges have a property which prohibits them from being processed and they remain acid. Thus they stay acid at every stage of their transit through the body and aggravate every part which they contact. All other citrus fruit are highly beneficial.

Vegemite is unsuitable because of its high salt content and Promite is unsuitable because of its high sugar content. Marmite is a compromise between the two. So if a person is going to be devastated without their vegemite, then they may use Marmite.

We do not use refined table salt, as this is an isolated chemical, sodium chloride. When this is put into the body it puts all the other mineral salts out of balance and so upsets the fluid and electrolyte system with sometimes dangerous results in the circulatory system and brain function. Also it usually has iodine added to it, a very important mineral for thyroid balance. But this, like everything else, should be obtained from natural sources and generally, the iodine added to table salt is not natural. It is alright to use sea salt as this contains natural mixtures of all the minerals and trace elements, including iodine, in the right balance. So a small amount of sea salt added to food is fine. It is also available mixed with ground vegetables for extra flavour and this is a very tasty seasoning called Vegisalt.

Alcohol is a problem for people who have a digestive enzyme deficiency because of the sugar, which is the basis of all alcoholic fermentation processes. So, before the actual alcohol hits the liver it has already caused a hypoglycaemic effect through the pancreas. This explains why so many so-called alcoholics go into blackouts and fits on a relatively small amount of alcohol. These people are not alcohol abusers, that is, they do not generally drink huge amounts of alcohol, but as soon as the first drink hits their system the brain chemistry changes and their normal responses no longer occur.

In other words, these people should never drink alcohol as their bodies will not process it and they have an immediate allergic response. Most alcohol is also full of chemicals and preservatives and is not naturally fermented in the bottle. It therefore remains very acid and it becomes like drinking a chemical cocktail, the results of which remain in our systems to interfere with our brain and liver processes long after the alcoholic effect has disappeared.

Soft drinks and cordials are unsuitable because they all contain sugar and most also contain preservatives, flavourings and colourings, even most of the flavoured mineral waters. Coca-Cola, milo, ovaltine, etc., all contain caffeine and sugar, some containing full cream milk products also, and artificial flavourings, colourings and preservatives.

Monosodium glutamate known as MSG, now called 'natural flavour enhancer No. 621' is a deadly liver poison and should be avoided. All processed food labels should be scanned for this insidious additive. It does not actually have a flavour of its own but brings out the flavour of the foods with which it is put. This is why it is so commonly used in Chinese food. These days many Chinese restaurants will cook without it if asked, but be sure to ask whether the food has been marinated in it or not.

MSG appears now mostly as 'natural flavour enhancer 621' and is added to most of the snacks that children love to eat, including corn chips and crisps, unless you purchase the unflavoured ones. It is also added to many otherwise healthy-looking biscuits, soups, gravy flavourings, even cakes. So please read the labels of everything you buy very carefully and make sure that your children are not ingesting this dangerous additive.

The artificial flavourings, colourings and preservatives set up many bad reactions in the liver and the kidneys, contributing together with chocolate and coffee to the formation of kidney stones and gravel. They also cause many bad skin problems and hyperactivity as the body tries to protect itself and eliminate as fast as possible through the skin thus trying to minimise the damage to the liver and kidneys.

The problem with milk and its products is that it contains large proportions of both fatty acids and milk sugars. If there is a digestive enzyme problem, then neither of these substances are going to be digested, thus setting them up as well known mucus producers. The reason that they produce mucus is that they are not digested initially by the pancreatic enzymes. So fermentation ensues, causing the mucus linings to throw out mucous to protect themselves from the acid thus produced.

Damage may than be caused to the lacteals, which produce the milk digesting enzymes from the tips of the many small villi which line the entrance to the gut, thus causing the milk sugars to remain undigested.

This also means that because the milk is not broken down properly the other properties of the milk cannot be absorbed. So drinking milk for its calcium content is a fallacy. Cow's milk is for baby cows and most species do not feed their young on milk for more than two years, by which time its properties should be able to be absorbed from other types of foods.

Soya milk and its products are a better alternative as long as it is not adulterated with oils and sugars, as are most of the readily available products on the market. Please read the labels carefully and remember that soy products, if processed properly and not merely soy isolates, are a whole protein and a starch. In other words, a whole food and should not be mixed with another protein, starch or fatty acid if there is a digestive enzyme problem. If they are not properly digested, their benefit, as a whole protein is lost because the nutrients aren't available to the body for assimilation. Use only a small amount at a time, carefully separated from other heavy foods and with digestive enzymes. This also applies to other soy products as well (crisps, mayonnaise, etc.), which are combined with other ingredients making them impossible to digest.

Soya products, tofu, tempeh and hatcho miso (this is the only one which contains no wheat or rice) are fermented, so are already partially digested making them easier for us to digest, if separated correctly in moderate quantities with digestive enzymes.

Soya sprouts are easier to digest but lose one of the

essential amino acids making them an incomplete protein.

Sour light cream seems to be alright as a transitionary product because it has most of the fat removed and is then cultured so most of the rest of the otherwise difficult to digest components are already partly pre-digested. This can be mixed with sweet or savoury, hot or cold foods and makes many dishes more appealing and interesting. It is a whole protein, but can be mixed with others in small quantities as the burden of digestion has been done already.

Food may be fried in lemon juice with a small amount of wheat-free, low-salt tamari with no fat or oil added at all. This makes the food very tasty and stops it from sticking to the pan long enough until the food produces its own juices from being heated.

The other meats which are alright during the period of transition, namely chicken, fish and game-meat, can also be cooked like this or grilled with lemon juice or baked in foil with lemon juice and tamari and herbs.

The reason that the skin must be taken off the chicken is that underneath and attached to that skin is a thin layer of fat, and this is where the chicken stores all of the drugs which it ingests during its life. Chickens produced on commercial farms are fed large quantities of hormones and antibiotics and should generally be avoided. However, occasionally in small quantities they do help the transition from being a daily meat eater to being a vegetarian. This transition in some people may take as long as 15 years, so don't worry if you think you can't do everything all at once. Every effort that you make will be more than you were doing before.

All vinegar except apple cider vinegar should be avoided as they contain malic acid, which is extremely harmful to our delicate and sensitive mucous linings, which by now you will probably have understood, are already under attack from many quarters. Apple cider vinegar, on the contrary, is an alkaline product and will help to cut the excess fatty acids in our system and act as a general cleanser. It is particularly helpful in clearing uric acid deposits and can be taken in arthritic situations as a drink: 2 tbsps apple-cider vinegar, 1 tspn organic honey, half a fresh squeezed lemon (small) and 1 tumbler of hot water. Dissolve all together. Can be drunk hot or cold any time. Try to obtain apple cider vinegar made from organically-grown apples and fermented naturally.

Foods Benefit to Most Bodies

Kelp. This is a natural source of all the minerals and trace elements we need including iodine (for thyroids) and lithium (for imbalance in our brain/ego pressure areas). This works very well with a zinc, magnesium and B6 supplement for relieving pre-menstrual tension, bloating and cramps.

Avocados. This wonderful fruit is a whole food and should be combined only with a green salad. They contain a small amount of protein and many minerals and vitamins and trace elements.

Lemons. A source of much vitamin C. Also a highly cleansing fruit which cuts through stored fatty acids and helps remove them from the system.

Mushrooms. These are another whole food. A whole protein together with many minerals vitamins and trace elements. Also a source of pancreatic enzymes. These may be eaten raw or cooked and mixed with other vegetables, starch or protein.

Bananas. A whole food. These are not fattening as long as they are not combined with any other food and if there is a digestive enzyme deficiency then an enzyme tablet may need to be taken after eating.

Eggs. Must be fresh, free-range from organically-fed chickens. May be used whole in mayonnaise or cooked as long as they are not fried. They are a whole food and should be combined only with a fresh salad. They only set up a cholesterol problem if combined with other fatty acids, proteins or starches.

Radishes. These contain a wonderful mixture of all food nutrients and are also very cleansing for the gall bladder.

Bee products. Royal Jelly, propolis, pollen and honey being the most commonly used. These all contain many nutrients, readily absorbed into the system. Propolis also acting as an antibiotic, especially to the anaerobic germs which live from our mouths, into our throats and right down through our digestive tracts.

Propolis is particularly useful for people with digestive enzyme problems who are very susceptible to infections in their mucous linings anywhere from the mouth right through to the anus. Pollen is particularly rich in zinc and other nutrients, which can negate hay fever and other allergic reactions from inhaled substances.

Parsley. This is another food which contains so many nutrients that we consider everybody should eat it by the bunch, not just as a garnish, which is how it is normally used. It contains large amounts of natural calcium, iron, Vit.C and Vit.A, together with protein and B vitamins and is particularly high in potassium.

Red capsicum. Particularly high in Vit.C and Vit.A. Also a small amount of protein and other minerals.

We should like you to know that for every disease that has already been mentioned, no matter how long-standing, something can be done to alleviate it, and in many cases completely reverse it. The choice is up to you.

---◆--- Chapter 7 ---◆---

THE ZINC LINK

Zinc is the main balancer of all the other minerals in our systems. It is necessary for proper protein usage, for proper sugar metabolism, for balanced hormonal functions, for fertility, for coping with stress and perhaps most important of all these, for proper functioning of the immune system. Also with vibrational healing we find that unless the minerals are balanced, and that means an adequate zinc absorption, only temporary advances can be made.

Our planet is largely depleted of natural zinc in the soil and so the food we eat cannot be relied upon to give us what we need, even if we are able to digest that food properly, which for most of us is not the case.

Until recently zinc was only considered a micro-nutrient, but it has now been realised that because it is involved in so many of the basic functions of the body, mind and spirit that we have to look again and re-evaluate our understanding of this vital food.

Emotional swings experienced in depression, pre-menstrual syndrome allergic reactions, etc., are also largely due to an imbalance of zinc which in turn imbalances other mineral mixtures and causes the body messengers (hormones) to dysfunction.

The zinc that is used for supplements must be from natural sources such as Royal Jelly or pollen granules. Synthetic zinc can be quite harmful to the whole body system as it is difficult to metabolise. Most people who have a zinc deficiency do so because they cannot metabolize natural zinc, it follows therefore that they are not going to be able to break down a chemical tablet to obtain synthesised zinc.

The following are some of the factors which interfere with human intake of zinc.

Zinc is water soluble and is easily leached from the soil by rain, which washes away the zinc salts, so that the plants are already deficient in zinc even when they are eaten raw. This also means that cooking the food in water is going to cause loss of zinc out of that food into the water which is then usually discarded.

Refining of food causes loss of zinc. White flour (and all its associated products) has lost nearly all of its zinc which is held in the fibrous parts, all of which are discarded in the refining process.

Zinc is available in red meat but in order to use it the meat has to be able to be digested. Most of us do not break the meat fibres down sufficiently to extract the zinc from them. We also have the same problem with nuts, as the fatty acids have to be broken down first in order to absorb the zinc and most of us do not manage that either.

There is zinc available in oysters in large concentrations but as they are also very high in cholesterol, ingesting large numbers of oysters is not recommended.

Mushrooms contain large amounts of zinc and also of the B vitamins. They are a whole vegetable protein and a source of digestive enzymes which help to absorb and use the zinc.

The safest readily absorbable source of natural zinc is pure, fresh Royal Jelly from the beehive, also pollen granules, freeze dried, contain an abundance of natural zinc. Royal Jelly not only contains large amounts of useable zinc, but also contains the whole range of B vitamins, the richest natural source of B5, pantothenic acid, small amounts of Vitamins A, C and E, many other minerals and trace elements. It is a natural antibiotic. Germs cannot live in Royal Jelly for more than a few minutes.

When zinc supplements are taken in a tablet form they should be a chelated product. This process combines the mineral with an amino acid, which it would normally have to be combined with in a digestive process. This process has already been accomplished and so this part of the digestion can be by-passed, thus ensuring that even if there is a digestive problem, the zinc is still going to be able to be absorbed. The body readily excretes any excess zinc.

These days the immune system requires huge amounts of natural zinc in order to function competently. Zinc and Vitamin A work very closely together (the Vit. A must also be from natural sources). Zinc and Vit. A work to combat pollution inside and outside the body, which is why they are now needed in such large quantities. These also work in very close relationship with Vit. C, Vit. B6, and magnesium.

Candida and Thrush

These are very much associated with zinc deficiencies. The candida feed on undigested starches and fatty acids mainly caused by a pancreatic enzyme deficiency and or over-indulgence of the above foods. This problem causes difficulties in sugar metabolism. The starches ferment causing acid to be formed, this aggravates the mucous linings of the digestive system and they pour out mucus to protect themselves.

Zinc and Vit.A are largely concerned with keeping these mucous linings healthy, so this constant onslaught of acids from the fermenting undigested food is a continuous drain on the zinc levels which are already depleted because of the extra demand for zinc at the sugar metabolism level.

The candida also consumes large amounts of Vit. B6, which works with the zinc on many levels, especially in the functioning of the immune system, and in the metabolism of starches and fatty acids. Vit. B6 depends on zinc being available in the system to perform nearly all its functions. It is very much involved in the brain chemistry of depression, in the formation of red blood cells, and in keeping the blood sugar balanced; none of which it can manage without adequate useable zinc.

When zinc and Vit. B6 levels are low or out of balance, sugar cravings set in, leading the person to overload on starches, thus making the problem even worse and giving the candida more of their favourite food. This often then leads to tiredness, depression and a very low immune system, encouraging infections, particularly of the mucous membrane system, which is already aggravated at this stage and ready to play host to any number of anaerobic germs (those germs which thrive without oxygen).

Herpes
Another dysfunction largely associated with zinc deficiency together with a deficiency of one of the essential amino acids (eight of which make up a whole protein) called L-Lysine.

Outbreaks of herpes, which is considered by experts to be a virus, generally happen during or immediately after times of great stress. In other words, when all the available zinc, which could be keeping the herpes virus at bay is being used up dealing with the external stress situation. Herpes also occurs when the diet is rich in sugary and or fatty foods.

Another occasion is when the available zinc will be used up coping with the stress on the sugar metabolism. As zinc has strong anti-viral properties, applications of this (as long as it is from natural sources) internally and externally will help to alleviate this problem. In the case of herpes the zinc works well with L-Lysine, Vit. B6, Vit.C.

The food separation chart should also be followed. This will ensure that all starches are properly digested and will therefore not aggravate the situation further. A herbal cream can be applied topically containing Solanum Nigrum.

Kidney Stones

Kidney stones can be caused by a number of occurrences within the digestive system, most of these being associated with zinc deficiencies. The absorption of protein requires zinc, and if this is deficient in the system, some of the protein components will be precipitated and crystallise around the kidney area, especially in the loopy areas of the very fine tubules. This can show early as stiffness in the lower back in the morning, gradually feeling better as the day wears on. The formation of the gravel or stones is also largely due to lack of absorption of Vit. B6 and magnesium which work very closely with zinc.

Natural supplementation of B6, magnesium and zinc can prevent the recurrence of kidney stones or gravel once they have been dispersed with homoeopathic and other natural treatments.

Pancreatic Enzyme Useability

Zinc and Vit. B6 are essential in the body's fat and starch metabolism, which begins with pancreatic enzyme production. Without proper metabolism at this elementary stage, very little absorption of any food can take place. This becomes a vicious circle because the essential zinc and B6 cannot be obtained from the food if it is not broken down in the first place. In other words, all body metabolism is impaired without adequate useable zinc and B6 in the system.

Digestive Disturbances – Constipation – Abdominal Pain
Because of the above-mentioned disturbance in the breakdown
of the food if there is a deficiency of useable zinc in the system,
bloating, constipation, abdominal pain, nausea, etc., may all occur.
The above symptoms can all be reversed with suitable food
separation and an adequate intake of useable zinc and associated
vitamins.

Cholesterol and Gall Bladder Problems
Because of the role which zinc plays in the fat metabolism, a
deficiency can cause the fatty acids to be half-processed and
sent through the system in an unsuitable form. This contributes
to the accumulation of cholesterol throughout the body or the
formation of gallstones and gravel which cause much aggravation,
inflammation and pain throughout the whole system.

Hypoglycaemia and Diabetes
Adequate zinc is essential for proper sugar metabolism,
deficiencies leading first to hypoglycaemia, and if unattended,
can eventually lead to age-onset diabetes where there is also a
pancreatic enzyme deficiency.

Eyesight
Poor eyesight onset can be largely due to a zinc deficiency. There
must be enough zinc and natural Vit. A in the system for good
eyesight to be maintained.

When the eyesight gradually starts getting more blurred,
focusing is harder and more concentration is needed to read, it's
time to look at our natural zinc intake. This can be one of our first
warning signs that our metabolism isn't all that it should be.

A healthy functioning eye contains large amounts of stored
zinc.

Pre-menstrual Syndrome, Infertility and Prostate Problems
After ovulation, a hormone called ceruloplasmin is released for about seven days before menstruation. This is composed largely of copper. The ratio between zinc and copper is very sensitive and this surge of copper into the system unbalances the whole mineral content of the body. This can lead to very unbalanced behaviour, also swelling of the breasts, ankles and stomach, backache, headache, pins and needles in hands or arms and impaired thyroid function. To re-balance this, large quantities of natural zinc and kelp are taken together with magnesium, B6 and essential fatty acids, particularly starflower, blackcurrant seed and linseed oils.

Infertility
Again we have to look at the zinc concentrations in the system, both of the male and the female. Both reproductive systems are hugely dependent on zinc. The sperm are made almost entirely of zinc. If the male is not absorbing enough of this out of his food, then the sperm are not going to be strong enough to make the long and arduous journey from the vagina to meet and fertilise the egg. A sperm count really does not tell us very much of relevance. We do not need to know how many there are; we need to know how much zinc they are composed of. Only one sperm is needed to fertilise the egg; the rest of them are necessary to break through the outer shell of the egg to let the fertilising sperm in.

If the fertile mucus in the vagina is deficient in zinc because of poor absorption from the food, then two problems are going to occur.

Firstly, the vaginal medium is going to be too acid as a result of the undigested fatty acids and starches fermenting. This acid will kill off all but the strongest of sperm. Secondly, if this vaginal medium is deficient in zinc, there is no food for the sperm to feed on as it travels on its long voyage.

The prostate gland suffers severely from lack of zinc. This can lead to pain and swelling and other discomfort. Zinc deficiency in males can lead to impotence, premature ejaculation and other associated disorders, which can be readily treated with adequate useable zinc and other natural means.

Chronic Fatigue Syndrome

Protein and carbohydrate metabolism are so dependant on sufficient zinc being available that when the body has to struggle on with an inadequate supply, the liver eventually begins to suffer from stress and overwork. At the same time as it is being asked to do extra work, it is being under-nourished and then the whole system breaks down.

This condition is now recognised as chronic fatigue syndrome. This is readily overcome by correct nutrition, rest and other body regeneration substances such as large quantities of Royal Jelly which contains more readily absorbed zinc than anything else, antioxidants such as Vit E., COQ10, lycopenes, grape seed extract and echinacea. The above treatment also applies to other liver degenerative diseases such as glandular fever, cancer and aids.

Skin and nail disorders

The skin needs plenty of zinc in the system together with adequate supplies of natural Vit. A and some amino acids in order to maintain its integrity. Zinc is a vital component of collagen which controls the skin's elasticity. Lack of zinc in the system can lead to psoriasis and other drastic skin conditions.

White spots in the nails are a sign of zinc deficiencies. It takes three months for a nail to grow from the cuticle to the top of the finger, so wherever the white spot is in the nail, the time of the zinc deficiency can be worked out. In women it will very often coincide with the monthly period. If a person has been under much stress, which uses up a great deal of zinc and other minerals, this is also likely to show up in the nail as a white spot or even a crosswise ridge. The malformation of toenails can also generally be attributed to an imbalance of systemic zinc.

Arthritis

An imbalance of the copper/zinc ratio is found in most cases of arthritis. When additional zinc is given many of the arthritic symptoms disappear, especially if given in a natural supplement such as Royal Jelly combined with other natural therapies.

In our research we have found that mental and emotional disorders are largely tied up with mineral imbalances and or deficiencies. Not only must all the minerals be present, in the right amounts, they must also be in a specific ratio to each other, which is different for each one and must also be in a specific ratio to many vitamins. In the case of mental and emotional disorders, the B vitamin group appears to be of the greatest importance. Here again, not only must all the B vitamins be present at the same time, they must be in a specific ratio to each other and to the minerals they work with, notably zinc.

All cells in the body must have these correct mixtures of minerals and vitamins or deficiencies will occur. Body fluids are also composed of cells which must have all the correct mixtures in order to join in the functional process of the whole organism. Nerve cells (neurones) pass their vital messages to each other through a medium called neuro-transmitter fluid. This is in fact a hormone.

If this fluid does not have the correct mineral mixtures, the message from one nerve cell to another either does not get across at all or gets distorted and a different or unbalanced message gets passed on, especially the emotional messages.

All hormones are very dependent on zinc for a correct balance. When emotional disturbances occur through lack of adequate minerals, nothing other than administration of natural minerals (zinc is always deficient in these cases) is going to re-balance that person. No known chemical treatment is going to effect a permanent cure for a zinc deficiency.

Pre-menstrual syndrome, chronic fatigue syndrome, schizophrenia, Alzheimer's disease, Parkinson's disease, multiple sclerosis, manic depression, imbalanced thyroid, anorexia nervosa and bulimia and obsessive behaviour, etc., all have their base roots in mal-absorption of minerals, notably zinc and B vitamins.

Some of the people suffering from any or all of the above disorders may indeed have had them from birth, as their body cells may have inherited toxic matter as part of their natural order. This means that the disorder itself is considered by that particular body to be its ordinary state, so the normal process of the body ridding itself of toxic waste does not occur. The body does not attempt to absorb any different mineral mixture other than that which it considers to be normal.

This inherited body pattern is very difficult to overcome but can be done with natural means, much determination and a lot of support from friends and/or family. It seems that these inherited body patterns cannot be overcome without great emotional support, thus proving that love has a pattern all of its own and can be involved in changing absolutely anything to its ultimate beauty.

Where the disorder has been acquired and not inherited, it is always possible to detoxify the system and restore the normal cell constituents by natural means and by the correct mineral and vitamin mixtures. Eventually, if the reason for the mal-absorption is recognised, the acquired body pattern can be reversed and maintained.

Spiritual

There are some types of work which we do requiring a higher or different rate of vibration than is used in normal day to day living. The involvement of zinc in these processes has proved to be of great interest.

If we as the facilitators of the energy that we are going to work with have a high concentration of natural zinc in our system, then we can access a fairly high vibration to work with. If the person we are going to work with also has high zinc levels, then the vibration that we can access together will be even higher.

The reason that we are seeking a higher (faster) vibration to play with is because when asking for esoteric information we can only access and receive according to the highest vibration which we are displaying ourselves. Information from a higher source than our vibration would not make sense to us or we would not use it correctly.

Source energy has the highest vibration and is not dependent on anything for its rate of vibration – it just is. We do find it difficult generally to receive completely unconditional love in its true spirit as our own vibration would rarely match it.

We have found that in large groups of meditative people the highest concentration of this 'source energy' vibration can be absorbed. The meditative process seems to transcend the ego (which generally lowers our vibratory rate) and allows us to join in the group energy. This uses up huge amounts of zinc as we lift our vibrations to meet that which we are receiving. When we leave the group energy, which is supporting us, we can suffer an extreme low unless we are taking Royal Jelly or some other natural zinc supplement. In these cases we have not found anything to surpass Royal Jelly. It seems to have an extremely high vibratory rate which our bodies can use immediately. If we have been meditating or working with a large group of people at an esoteric level for a prolonged period of time, then when we return to so-called normal life the degree of zinc deficiency can be pronounced. This may often produce symptoms of chronic fatigue syndrome that takes some time to recover from. If the problem is not recognised or understood, recovery may not happen very readily.

The vibration of tobacco particularly and the actual physical use of it causes huge amounts of zinc to be lost from the system. Physically, smoking of tobacco leaves cadmium in the system which throws the zinc out. Cadmium is also produced in large quantities out of factory chimneys, so people who live or work in or near those kind of factories are constantly having the zinc leached out of their systems.

We have found it interesting that many people involved in esoteric work smoke tobacco and appear to have low zinc levels. It seems that they are deliberately (maybe unconsciously) keeping their vibratory levels lower as they possibly have a higher level than most people to start with and the information that they are accessing just doesn't fit in with the world they find themselves living in. There can be no excuse for prolonging this habit. Let us take full responsibility for being here now in a body and access the highest vibration that we possibly can. So the light can shine out through every cell in our body and not be darkened or completely extinguished by such a deliberate and premeditated process as ingesting tobacco.

How can the esoteric information these people are giving us be balanced and true and whole if they and their body systems are not? It seems that with the ability to collect and use the Royal Jelly now available, we have the chance to lift ourselves to a higher understanding of ourselves and what we are here for. This in turn gives a chance for the world to become a place of balance and harmony as we reflect our internal condition to our external environment.

---— ◆ —— Chapter 8 —— ◆ —---

REGENERATION

When we first change our food and drink, we are going to experience cleansing and healing. It is absolutely necessary during this time to get as much rest as possible. During the healing and cleansing stages, enormous amounts of minerals and energy are used up to facilitate these processes. If the person does not rest, the problems will take a long time to clear up and they will be tired most of the time. It is also very important to keep as warm as possible as this also uses up a lot of energy and minerals.

A small amount of gentle exercise may be taken such as half an hour walking, preferably not in a cold wind and not in traffic. Ten minutes on a rebounder is also okay, but no longer, and half an hour swimming as long as the water is warm. This amount of exercise may be taken daily just to keep the lymph and the circulation going to help with the cleansing, but any more than this and the vital minerals and energy we need for the cleansing and rebuilding will be lost.

After a few weeks, when the person begins to wake up and feels like leaping out of bed and singing and going for a run before breakfast, then the re-oxygenation of the body can really begin.

Oxygen is what we need urgently inside and outside our systems to burn up and take away the rubbish that we have accumulated in our deep tissues and to combine with the dangerous free radicals in our systems to take them out of the body. We can live for at least six weeks without food and possibly three weeks without water, but we can only survive three minutes without oxygen.

As our bodies are made up mainly of water and oxygen, it stands to reason that we are going to reap the most benefit from obtaining our oxygen supplies around or near water. Sparkling mountain streams, broad flowing rivers, and best of all – the sea.

Most of us do not breathe properly. Every part of our system requires oxygen for proper functioning. Without it we become clogged up and sluggish, creating dangerous cancerous situations within our minds and our bodies. So, first of all we have to learn to breathe properly, we have to learn to take the life-breath or 'chi' into our systems, circulate it and remove the old used-up breath. If we do not breathe out properly, then we are holding old toxic rubbish in our systems and that again causes a dangerous situation.

Yoga and tai chi are excellent for learning not only how to breathe in and out properly, but also how to mobilise the life-energy around the entire system.

We cannot stress enough how all degenerative diseases have come about, not only through improper digestion, but also through lack of complete oxygenation of the system at the same time. Any diseased cell needs to be combined with oxygen to assist it out of the system. A cell does not become diseased if it is properly nourished and receives enough oxygen.

Oxygen drops are now available at most good health food stores. These should be used in very small doses to start with, as the cleansing will be too uncomfortable if too many toxins are released at once. The dose can gradually be increased and may then be taken in pure water which has been red solarised. That is, water which has been exposed to sunlight in a red glass container for at least 24 hours. This greatly increases the oxygen and the energy giving properties of the water.

When the cleansing is well under way, a proper exercise regime should be worked out and maintained. Aerobic exercise is good as long as the teacher is well trained and the person starts off with gentle stretching and low impact. For most of us it is not necessary to progress beyond low impact as this gives all the circulation, stretching and oxygenation that we would need in normal circumstances without using up too many of our other valuable minerals. If we go into a really heavy aerobic routine, then we will need to supplement our minerals and amino acids to keep up with our output. Remember, any supplements that we take should always be natural.

Royal Jelly is always useful and echinacea has properties which allow it to rapidly help in oxygenation of our systems. We should build up our exercise to about 45 minutes three times a week or 20 minutes daily.

The most important part of this process is the under-standing that this change of food and consequently of lifestyle is not just a diet or a temporary activity. It is a commitment to give ourselves the best quality of life for the remainder of the time that we spend in the body we now inhabit. This undertaking requires dedication, determination and sensitivity. These qualities are available to all of us if we have the courage to look within and learn to trust our own knowing.

We have had great fun playing with the food and have discovered many wonderful and exotic ways of presenting healthy food, which looks, tastes and smells extremely inviting.

—◆—— Chapter 9 ——◆—

RECIPES

The following recipes are suggestions on ways in which the food may be mixed to give some variety to meals. They were not handed to us carved in stone tablets on a fiery mountain, so feel free to change by addition or subtraction any ingredients to suit your taste, mood, and most importantly, your digestion.

With any of the vegetable or salad dishes not containing starch, protein or fatty acid, you may add fish, chicken, tofu, rice, pasta, etc., if you wish. Check the combinations and modify accordingly. Vegetables may be steamed, stuffed, baked boiled, fried (not in oil, butter, etc.) in any combination of taste, texture or colour with herbs and spices for distinctive flavour. Express your creativity and not mediocrity in cooking for your being.

If you wish to combine more than one dish make sure that the resulting combination only contains:

One starch or one protein or one fatty acid.

In all the recipes please note that:
- Quantities are for 2-4 people, depending on appetite.
- Tamari is wheat-free and low salt.

- Salt refers to seasalt, rocksalt or vegesalt only.
- Freshly ground black pepper where possible.
- Oil is cold pressed, the lighter the oil the better, i.e., grape seed.
- Oil is not to be heated but may be poured unheated over hot vegetable dishes, which do not contain other proteins, starches or fatty acids.
- Herbs are fresh where possible.
- Curry or other powders are without fillers, which generally tend to be some type of starch and usually more than one kind. Canned tomatoes, etc., where required are to be without sugar and minimal salt.
- Tuna, or other canned fish, in brine or tomato sauce only. *Not oil.*
- Chicken, turkey and eggs to be free-range.
- Vinegar is always apple-cider vinegar.
- Frying is done dry in a non-stick pan/wok or either in tamari or some lemon.
- The best type of cooking utensils are stainless steel as the others tend to leave deposits in the cooking which are harmful to the stomach linings.
- Capsicums and apples are always of the red varieties as the green types contain salicylic acid which eats away the stomach lining.
- Eggplant – Pre-cooking preparation: Slice the eggplant leaving the skin intact, place in a flat container and liberally salt. Cover with flat tray, place weight on top (enough to press the slices but not to squash) and leave for a few hours, occasionally draining off the excess liquid. Rinse eggplant to get rid of salt and pat dry on a towel.

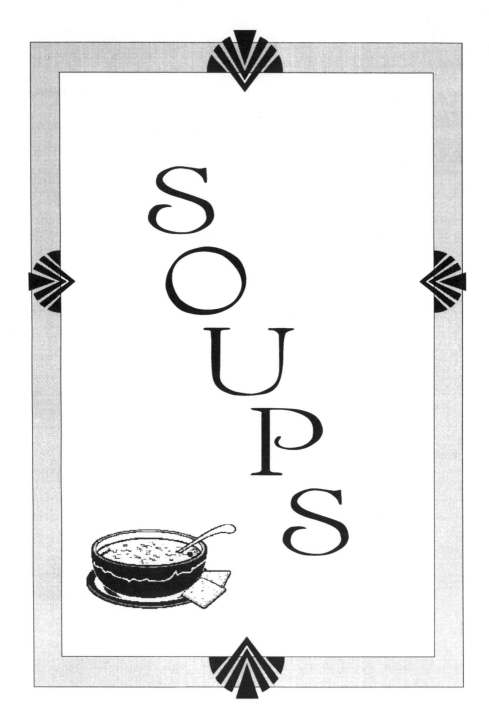

SOUPS

Smoked Salmon Tomato Soup

100-200 g smoked salmon   1 onion
2 tspns fenugreek powder   2 kg tomatoes
2 cloves garlic all roughly chopped   2 tspns cayenne powder
salt & pepper to taste
½-¾ cups coriander & parsley, finely chopped
water (use as necessary for the consistency you want)

Place all ingredients, except the salmon, into pot and bring to the boil. Simmer for 10-15 min, add the salmon, puree with hand blender and simmer for a further 10 min.

Bill's Tomato Soup

This is an easy to make soup for that cool winter evening after a long day at work.

1½ lt tomato juice (roughly the juice of 1-2 kg tomatoes)
½ cup parsley roughly chopped
2 tbsps finely chopped basil   2-3 tbsps tamari
salt & pepper to taste   2 tspns dry coriander
1 tspn paprika

Mix all ingredients in large pot, bring to boil, then simmer for 20-30 min.

Chilled Double Soup

This wonderful combination of green and red soups in the onebowl pleases your sense of sight as well as taste.

Cucumber

2 continental or Lebanese cucumbers, peeled
1 spring onion, thinly sliced
½ cup sour light cream   salt & pepper to taste
¼ cup fresh mint, chopped   pinch cumin

Capsicum

3 large red capsicums
2 spring onions, sliced
1 tspn paprika
1 tspn ground cumin
2-4 tomatoes, peeled, seeded and chopped
2 tspns fresh coriander roughly chopped

Cut cucumbers in half lengthways, remove seeds, sprinkle with salt; stand for 30 min. Rinse cucumbers under cold water, drain and pat dry. Blend cucumbers and sour light cream until smooth. Stir in mint, cumin and spring onion.

Season with salt and pepper. Transfer to jug, cover and refrigerate for about 1 hour. Quarter capsicums, grill skin-side up until skin blisters and blackens. Peel away skin and roughly chop. Blend capsicums, tomatoes, extra cumin and spring onions until smooth. Stir in coriander and paprika.

Season with salt and pepper and thin if necessary though we do not want it too thin. Transfer to jug, cover and then refrigerate for about 1 hr. Pour both soups into each serving dish from opposite sides, at the same time, so that you have two distinct halves. Garnish with capsicum and fresh herbs. Looks and tastes exquisite.

Indian Cucumber Soup

2 cucumbers peeled and chopped	water
1 cup seed cheese	½ tspn ground cumin
¼ cup finely chopped parsley	1 eschallot finely chopped

Blend ingredients together, adding water until smooth. Garnish with a little fresh dill or chives and serve at room temperature.

Gaspachio (Cold Tomato and Vegetable Soup)

6 medium tomatoes	500 ml water
½ capsicum	½ - 1 stick celery
dash of tamari	pinch of coriander powder
pinch of turmeric powder	1 cup mixed herbs

Roughly chop all ingredients together but do not puree as the soup needs to have that rough quality about it. Place in fridge and chill for half hour to 1 hour. Makes a beautiful summer entree.

Chickpea Soup

1½ cups chickpeas	1 carrot
1 large stick celery	1 onion
salt & pepper to taste	
1 tbsp tomato paste or 1 large tomato, pulped	

Soak the chickpeas overnight in cold water for about 12 hours. Wash well then boil in 2 litres of water for approximately 2 hours. If necessary add extra water to achieve desired consistency.

In an other pot cook the vegetables in a little water with the tomato or tomato paste then mix with the chickpeas.

Grilled Mediterranean Soup

4-6 medium tomatoes   3 large cloves of garlic
2 onions, sliced   basil & mint to taste
2 red capsicums, seeded & sliced   salt & pepper to taste

For this soup the tomatoes do not need to be peeled as all the ingredients will be pureed. Quarter the tomatoes and place under griller together with the capsicum, garlic, onion and 1 red capsicum. Cook until they start to char and blister (this will depend on your taste for charred vegies), then blend with the herbs and salt and pepper. You may extend the soup with some vegetable stock or tomato puree. Serve heated or chilled as an entree or main meal.

Creamy Golden Carrot Soup

1 kg carrots, grated   3 cloves garlic, crushed
1 tspn fresh ginger, grated   2 onions, sliced
1 cup green beans, chopped   1 tspn tomato paste
3 tbsps apple cider vinegar   coconut milk to taste
1 red capsicum, finely chopped   2 tspns cumin
1 tbsp mild curry powder   2 tspns turmeric
salt & pepper to taste

Fry onions, garlic and ginger in vinegar until browned then add some water and the carrots. Simmer for 5 min. then add more water, spices, coconut milk and rest of ingredients and simmer for 1 hour. If desired puree to give creamy texture.

Potato Cauliflower Soup

6 potatoes, steamed until slightly soft

2 cups cauliflower, chopped	3 cloves garlic, chopped
1 onion, chopped	3 squash, sliced
1 red capsicum, chopped	1 zucchini, sliced
2 tbsps tamari	6 cups water

1 cup red cabbage, finely chopped

1 cup basil, parsley, coriander, chopped

Sauté onion and garlic, slowly over a low heat, in a pot with the tamari until the onion is translucent. Add the rest of the vegetables stir for a while then add water and potato that has been pureed separately using one of the cups of water. Bring to the boil then turn heat down and simmer for 30-40 min. If desired you may then puree before serving. Garnish with chopped herbs and paprika.

Pumpkin Soup

1 medium or large pumpkin, peeled & chopped roughly

2 onions, chopped roughly	1 tspn crushed garlic
2 carrots, chopped	½ stick celery, chopped
2 tbsps apple cider vinegar	½ cup tamari
250 g button mushrooms	1 lt water
3 tspns cumin powder	3 tspns curry powder
salt & pepper to taste	¼ tspn nutmeg
3 tspns paprika (hot or sweet)	1 vegetable stock cube

1 tspn crushed or finely grated ginger

Sauté the onions with all the spices, ginger and garlic over a low heat while you cut up the remaining vegetables and pumpkin. When the onion has become translucent add the tamari and vinegar and stir.

Put all of the other ingredients into the pot, add water, bring to the boil then reduce heat and simmer until tender. Puree in blender and serve garnished with a sprig of parsley. (The tamari may be substituted with 1 good tbsp of hatcho miso. This is the one with no rice, etc.)

Carrot & Celery Stir-fry Soup

½ kg carrots, roughly chopped
150 g oyster mushroom
100 g green beans, chopped
1 yellow zucchini, sliced
1 cup red cabbage, shredded
¼ cup fresh sage, coriander roughly chopped

1 red capsicum, chopped
1 onion, chopped
salt & pepper to taste

Steam carrots and celery until tender (add the coriander to the water so that when it steams, the coriander flavours the carrot and celery. This is a good way to use old herbs that are about to go off). Puree the carrot and celery, using 2 cups of water strained from the steamer, add the sage and simmer over a low heat while you prepare the rest of the ingredients. Stir-fry the remaining ingredients until browned then add the puree and simmer together for 5 min. Can be used as an entree or main dish.

Red Lentil Soup

1 large onion, roughly chopped
1-2 cloves garlic, crushed
2 large carrots grated
1 bay leaf

1 tspn dry thyme
250 g red lentils
2 tbsps tamari
1½ lt water

2 tbsps parsley   3 tbsps tomato paste
handful shredded cabbage

Stir-fry onion, garlic, thyme and carrots for a few minutes, then add remaining ingredients. Bring to boil, cover and simmer for 40 min. To really bring out the best flavour allow to cool then reheat.

Note: You may use tomato paste instead of the fresh tomato but if you do, add it at the end as the salt in the tomato paste will cause the lentils not to boil.

Broccoli Soup

1 head broccoli & 1 head cauliflower, flowerets
1 cup chicken stock (or water and miso)
1 capsicum   1 zucchini, sliced
1 onion, sliced   250 g beanshoots
1 tomato, chopped   1 tspn cumin
salt and pepper to taste   dash cayenne

Steam broccoli then puree in blender with broth (or water and miso). Season and gently heat with the rest of the ingredients except the beanshoots which you add just before serving.

Carrot & Coriander Soup

2 carrots, sliced   1 onion, rings
2 eschallots, sliced   2 cloves garlic, crushed
1 medium capsicum, sliced   1 tbsp miso
4 cups water   1 cup chopped coriander

Lightly steam carrots and puree in blender with the coriander and add some water if needed. Add to the other vegetables in water and bring to boil then simmer for about 10-15 min.

Curried Vegetable Soup

Curry
1 onion, finely chopped
1 tspn chilli paste
1 tsp. garam masala
3 cups water

2 cloves garlic
3 tbsps curry powder
2 tbsps tomato paste

Dry stir-fry onion, garlic, curry and garam masala. Add tomato paste, chilli and water and simmer 10 to 15 min.

Vegetables
100 g green beans, halved
2 medium zucchini sliced
1 tbsp tamari
250 g button mushrooms, halved

2 eschallots, sliced
1 carrot, sliced
1 tbsp vinegar

Chop vegetables and stir-fry with tamari and vinegar until lightly cooked. Add vegetables, and extra water if desired, to curry and stir for a few min. then serve.

Leek and Cauliflower Soup

1 small cauliflower, cut into flowerets
2 leeks, chopped
4 cups water

2 tbsps tamari
salt & pepper to taste

Cook leeks until transparent. Add remainder of ingredients and bring to boil. Reduce heat and simmer for 10 min. May be pureed.

Potato and Cauliflower Soup

4 med. potatoes, peeled and cubed
6 flowers of cauliflowers, chopped
4 cloves garlic, crushed
½ cup shredded red cabbage
¼ cup red capsicum, chopped
1 tspn Chinese 5-spice
1 tspn garam masala
1 tbsp tamari
1 cup freshly chopped parsley, mint, coriander

salt & pepper
dash hot paprika
1 onion, finely chopped
3 grated carrots, sliced
1 eschallot, sliced
1 tspn cumin
1 tspn hatcho miso
1 tbsp vinegar

Place all ingredients in soup pot fill with water and simmer for 30 min. Mash with potato masher and simmer another 15 min.

Mushroom Soup

250 g mushrooms of choice, halved
1 medium onion, finely chopped
1 red capsicum, chopped

4 cups water
1 tspn cumin
1 tspn fenugreek powder

Place all ingredients in saucepan and bring to boil then simmer until mushrooms sink to the bottom of the pan. You may leave the mushrooms whole or puree the soup for a richer thicker consistency.

Tomato Soup With Basil

1 cup celery finely chopped
2 medium leeks, finely chopped
2 kg tomatoes, roughly chopped
1 cup water

3 cloves garlic, crushed
3 tbsps basil
2 tbsps tamari

In a large saucepan add garlic, leeks, celery, water and simmer for about 10 min. Add tomatoes, basil and simmer for further 20 min.

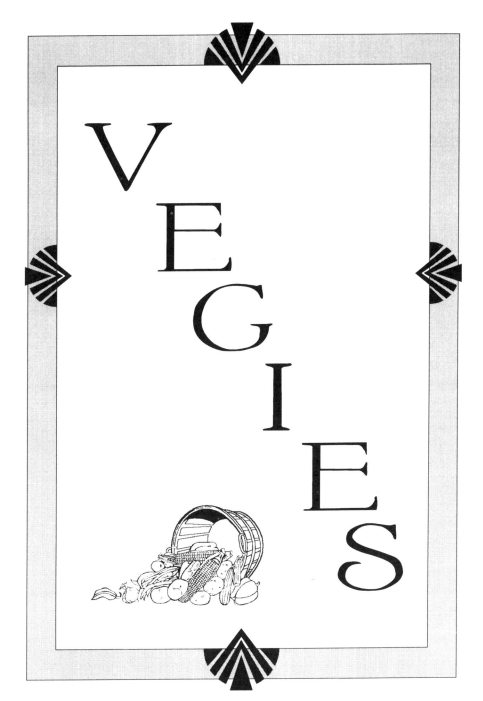

VEGIES

Risotto Rice

300-375 g brown rice
1 cup broccoli
1 tspn garlic, crushed
1 carrot cut into small cubes
1 onion, finely chopped
2 golden squash, thinly sliced
2 tspns paprika (sweet or hot)
1 cup capsicum, cut into small cubes
1 cup stock or stock cube (may be chicken or vegetable)
boiling water available

1 tbsp mixed herbs
1 tspn tumeric
1 tspn ginger, crushed
1 cup cauliflower
salt & pepper to taste
celery to taste

Slowly sauté onions with the herbs and spices until the onions are translucent. Add the rest of the vegetables and lightly stir-fry for a few min. Add the rice, and enough boiling water and stock to cover the rice and vegetables. Cover pan or pot with lid and bring mixture to boil. Turn down to a medium heat and simmer. Periodically check and add more water as it is absorbed by the rice. Cook until rice is done. You may make this dish as moist as you want by varying the amount of water added.

Felafel

2½ cups chick peas, soaked overnight
½ bunch of parsley
2 tspns cumin powder
½ tspn hot paprika
salt & pepper to taste

juice of 1 lemon
1 tspn coriander powder
4 cloves garlic, peeled
½ cup water

Using a food processor put all ingredients (except water) in together and process until it becomes a paste. Add the water slowly until you get the right consistency. Spoon mixture into a non-stick pan and fry each side for about 5 min. until golden brown. Serve with wonderful relishes, chutneys or hommous as per recipes in this book. May be frozen uncooked until required.

Potato Wedges

8-10 med. washed potatoes (cut into 8 pieces, or fries)
¼ cup tamari
1 tspn garlic, crushed   1 tspn hot paprika
salt & pepper to taste   1 tbsp mixed herbs

Preheat oven to 200° C. Put potatoes onto tray lined with foil and brush with mixture. Bake until potatoes are cooked (basting twice more during cooking) and browned.

Mexican Beans

2 cups kidney beans   ¼ cup tomato paste
1 tbsp fresh ginger   1 tspn cumin powder
1 tspn coriander powder   1 tspn fenugreek powder
 salt & pepper to taste   1 tspn chilli powder
1 large onion, roughly chopped
350 mls tomato sauce
4-5 cloves garlic, finely chopped

Soak beans overnight then cook for about one hour (no salt), drain most of the water. Add the remaining ingredients, cook for about 15-25 min. and leave to cool slightly before serving. May be frozen and reheated.

Coconut Korma Cauliflower

250 ml coconut milk
1 tbsp mild Korma Curry powder
½ a cauliflower in small flowerets
2 handfuls green beans, roughly chopped
finely chopped tarragon, mint, coriander, parsley

2 small carrots, sliced
2 tspns cinnamon
1 onion, thinly sliced

Cook vegetables and spices in half a cup of water in a well-sealed pot over a medium heat until nearly done. Add the coconut milk, stir and close lid. Allow to sit for 5 min. then serve.

Marinated Mushrooms

250 g button mushrooms
1 clove garlic, crushed
1 tbsp vinegar
salt & pepper to taste

½ tspn lemon rind
4 tbsps oil
1 tbsp mint

Mix mushrooms and garlic in a bowl. Add the remaining ingredients to a jar and mix well, pour over the mushrooms and allow to sit in the fridge for about 2 hrs. Stir occasionally. Remove from fridge, drain and serve (keep the marinade for something else).

Spicy Lentils and Vegetables

1 cup red lentils
juice of ½ lemon
2 cloves garlic, finely chopped
1 tspn each ground ginger, turmeric, coriander & cumin
1 cup green beans, cut into short lengths
4-5 fresh tomatoes, peeled & quartered

1 onion, sliced
salt & pepper to taste

2 cups vegetable stock or dissolved vegetable stock cube
1 bunch coriander washed and chopped

Fry onion gently in large saucepan until tender then add garlic, ginger and spices and stir-fry for 1-2 min. Add lentils, beans, tomatoes, stock, salt and pepper. Bring to the boil, cover, then reduce heat and cook gently for about 20 min. or until lentils and vegetables are cooked and the liquid has been absorbed.

Scatter lemon juice and coriander over the vegetables and serve hot with your favourite relish or chutney.

Cabbage Goulash

½ small cabbage, finely shredded	½ tspn mixed herbs
1 onion, thinly sliced	pinch nutmeg
2 carrots, diced	2 zucchini, sliced
½ tspn caraway seeds	600 ml tomato juice
freshly chopped parsley	½ tspn paprika

Sauté onion and carrot in pan over a medium heat until the onion is translucent. Add zucchini and cabbage and cook for a further 10 min. Add paprika, caraway seeds, herbs, nutmeg and tomato juice. Cover and simmer for 10 min. or until the vegetables are just tender. Spoon the goulash into a dish, drizzle lightly with sour light cream and sprinkle with parsley.

Tomato and Onion Pie

4 ripe tomatoes	3 large onions
salt & pepper	½ cup chopped herbs
1 cup of breadcrumbs (see notes on bread)	

Core the tomatoes and slice. Peel the onions and slice, push into rings. Alternate the layers of tomatoes and onions in a dish, lightly sprinkling each tomato layer with salt and pepper. Mix the bread with herbs and sprinkle on top of the tomatoes and onion. Bake at 175°C for 40 min.

Almond Mushroom Surprise

2 small onions, chopped fine
4 sprigs parsley finely cut
25 g (½ cup) almond meal
handful snow peas, halved
dash hot paprika
tbsp apple cider vinegar

1 kg mushrooms, sliced
1 red capsicum, sliced
1 eschallot, chopped
½ cup hot water
dash tamari1
salt & pepper to taste

2 tspns each of cumin, cinnamon & fenugreek powder

Place onions in pan with the spices, mix well and cook over high heat until onions start to sizzle. Add tamari and apple cider vinegar then turn down heat to low and simmer. Mix in capsicum, mushrooms and snow peas. Cook over low heat until mushrooms have released liquid then sprinkle over almond meal, and when thoroughly mixed in, add water as desired. Simmer for 5 min., stir in parsley. Serve surrounded with crisp shredded lettuce.

Potato Patties

6 medium sized potatoes
1 red capsicum
½ cup broccoli
½ cup herbs, to own taste

2 medium carrots
½ an onion
½ cup cauliflower
spices to taste

Roughly chop potatoes and vegetables and steam until tender

(potatoes may also be boiled.). Combine the potatoes with the vegetables and herbs and spices in a large bowl and mash using a potato masher. When they are all mixed together make into patties and fry lightly in a non-stick pan until each side is crispy.

Potato Gratin

3 large potatoes, skins on and thinly sliced
1½ tspns mustard of choice
450 ml vegetable stock or use stock cube
1 tbsp fresh tarragon
150 ml sour light cream

Preheat oven to 190°C. Layer potatoes in a casserole dish seasoning well with salt and pepper between the layers. Mix together mustard, tarragon, cream and stock together and pour over the potatoes. Cover with foil and bake in the oven for 1 hour. Remove the foil and cook for a further 25 min.

Aromatic Stuffed Peppers

2.5 cm piece fresh ginger root, freshly grated
1 tbsp black or brown mustard seeds
105 g quick cook brown rice   2 cloves garlic, crushed
1 tspn ground coriander   250 ml vegetable stock
8 medium capsicums, de-seeded   1 tspn cumin seeds
1 green chilli pepper, finely chopped   1 tspn ground paprika

Slice tops off and keep fresh coriander, roughly chopped
Preheat the oven to 180°C.
    Add the mustard and cumin seeds, chilli pepper, coriander and paprika and cook over a low flame until the spices and seeds

become aromatic. Add the ginger and garlic and dry-fry for a further 3 min. until the vegetables are soft. Add the rice, mix well and cook for 2 min. Pour in the stock and cook, uncovered until rice is cooked. Add extra liquid if needed (some white wine if you want).

When the rice is cooked add the coriander leaves then fill each pepper, replace the top and bake in the oven for 20 min.

Zucchini and Tomato Pie

2 onions, sliced
1 kg zucchini, sliced
2 cloves garlic, chopped
1 tbsp tomato paste
6 tomatoes, skinned (see appendix)

Topping
1 kg potatoes, boiled and mashed
4 eschallots, finely chopped

Place onions and zucchini in pan and fry for 10 min. Add garlic, tomatoes and tomato paste, salt and pepper to taste. Simmer for 5 min. and place into ovenproof dish. Mix the potatoes with the eschallots and spoon over zucchini mix. Cook in preheated oven at 200°C for 20-30 min.

Mediterranean Beans

1½ cups black-eyed beans	4 cups water
1 onion, chopped	1 bay leaf
½ cinnamon stick, halved	1 red capsicum
250 g mushrooms, chop if large	4 cloves garlic, halved

400 g tomatoes, chopped
2 tspns ground coriander
1 tspn whole cumin seeds

1 tspn ground cumin
½ tspn ground turmeric
salt & pepper to taste

Wash then drain beans and place in saucepan with water, half the onion and bay leaf. Bring to the boil, cover and simmer for 10 min. Turn off heat and leave to stand for 1 hour. Bring back to boil and simmer for 20 min. or until beans are tender. Remove from heat and set aside.

Heat non-stick pan and fry cinnamon stick and cumin seeds until fragrant. Add garlic, remaining half of the onion and pepper strips and cook gently. Then add mushrooms and tomatoes with the remaining spices. Simmer gently for 10 min.

Drain beans, reserve liquid, then add to vegetables and simmer uncovered for a further 10 min. Add the remaining ingredients and bring to the boil, then simmer over a low heat, stirring frequently.

Stir-Fry Vegetables with Spicy Skim Milk Feta Sauce

4 medium-sized carrots
½ large zucchini, thinly sliced

4 medium onions, sliced
2 bok choy, sliced

Sauce
4 tspns paprika
2 tbsps cumin
4 tspns aniseed powder
200 g skim milk feta

2 tspns hot paprika
2 tspns onion powder
3 tspns ginger powder
water

Slice carrots into 5 cm thin fingers and put in pan with onions. Dry fry over a low heat until they start to 'sweat' and continue to cook for a further 10 min. Add the other vegetables and turn up the heat to a medium flame and leave to cook.

In the meantime add the spices to a non-stick pot and heat until they become aromatic. Add the fetta cheese and allow to slowly melt, stirring constantly. Mix in enough water to make the sauce as thin as required and stir continuously. If necessary whisk to get out any lumps. Add the sauce to the vegetables and mix together. Serve with a garnish of fresh herbs.

Baked Pumpkin

½ medium butternut pumpkin, de-seeded
salt & pepper to taste

Stuffing
2 sticks celery, finely chopped
4 spring onions, finely chopped
2 cloves garlic, crushed

¼ cup parsley
1 tbsp tamari
salt & pepper to taste

Cut the pumpkin into half, spoon out the seeds and bake on a non-stick tray at 190°C for about 45 min. or until tender. Leaving 2 cm of flesh in the skin. Scoop out the remaining pumpkin flesh and chop roughly. Mix with the other ingredients and place mixture back into shell. Bake at 180°C for 15 min.

May be topped with onion sauce and served with a sprout salad.

Cabbage Roll

2 cabbage leaves per person (soft green leaves)
1 capsicum red, chopped
6 mushrooms, chopped
2 cups cooked brown rice

1 onion, chopped
1 stick celery, chopped
salt & pepper to taste

Sauce
400 g tin tomatoes, pureed
1 tspn basil
2 cloves garlic, chopped

Pour boiling water over cabbage leaves to soften them. Drain and cut out hard pieces of stalks. Mix other ingredients together and place a portion on each cabbage leaf. Roll up the leaves and fold in the ends. Mix all the sauce ingredients and pour one third of the mixture into casserole dish. Place rolls in dish with final fold on bottom. Pour on the remainder of the sauce. Cover and bake in a moderate oven for 30 min.

Arrange on dish and surround with sprouts and finely shredded capsicum and cucumber.

Carrot and Potato Bake

6 medium carrots, chopped
3 medium potatoes, chopped
1 medium onion, finely chopped
1 eschallot, finely chopped
1 stick celery, finely chopped
2 medium onions, cut into rings

2 cloves garlic, crushed
1 capsicum red, diced
1 tspn nutmeg
1 tbsp parsley
salt & pepper to taste

Steam carrots and potatoes until they are tender enough to mash. Add the onion, celery, capsicum, eschallot and salt and pepper. Mix together and place in a shallow ovenproof dish.

Sauté onion rings for 3 min. in 2 tbsps tamari and place on top of vegetables. Sprinkle parsley and nutmeg over the top and bake in moderate oven for 15-20 min. Grilled Herb Tomatoes are an excellent addition to this dish with slices of fresh cucumber, sprouts and shredded greens.

Cashew Stir-Fry

1 cup carrots, sliced
1 onion, sliced
1 zucchini, sliced
2 cloves garlic, chopped
1 tspn cumin
1 tspn fenugreek
1 cup cauliflower broken into flowerets

1 cup cashews
1 capsicum red, diced
4 eschallot, chopped
120 g mushrooms, sliced
salt & pepper to taste
2 tbsps tamari

First lightly heat the cashews, in 1-2 tbsps tamari, until they make a hollow sound when tapped. Allow to cool while preparing the rest.

Dry-fry the garlic and onion with the spices in tamari until they start to brown. Add the cauliflower, carrots and zucchini and cook for 5 min. Stir continuously to prevent burning. When they are just becoming tender, mix in the remainder of the vegetables and stir until they are all cooked. Mix in the cashews and serve with a crisp garden salad containing no other protein, starch, or fatty acid.

Chinese Cabbage

2 cloves garlic, chopped
1 tspn ginger, grated
1/3 cabbage, shredded finely
1 tspn paprika

Sauté garlic in a quarter cup of water for 2 min., then add cabbage, ginger and paprika. Stir for 2 min., cover and cook for 4 min. on low heat. May be served with either Sweet and Sour Stir-fry or Minted Mushrooms.

Coconutty Vegetable Curry

2 onions, sliced
1 tbsp green curry paste
225 g mushrooms
fresh coriander to taste, chopped
1 tspn miso, dissolved in hot water

4 cloves garlic, crushed
1 lemon, juice
1 knob of ginger, grated
400 ml lite coconut milk
1 kg mixture of vegetables

Cook the onion, ginger and garlic in the lemon juice, miso and a little water until the onion is very soft. Add the coconut milk, curry paste, coriander and vegetables and cook on a low heat for about 1 hour. Add the mushrooms and cook an extra 15 min. Ideal served with Spaghetti Marrow which has been steamed.

Grilled Herb Tomatoes

1 tomato per person
lemon juice
basil, mint, oregano, freshly chopped

salt & pepper to taste
tamari

Halve the tomatoes and spike them with a fork ensuring that the skin is not broken. Add salt and pepper, top with the herbs and pour over the tamari and lemon juice. Wrap the tomato halves in foil and grill for 10 min. under a medium flame or bake in the oven. An excellent addition to Carrot and Potato Bake.

Steamed Minted Vegetables

½ cauliflower, in flowerets
1 head broccoli, in flowerets

½ bunch mint
1 carrot, sliced

Place the mint on the bottom of the top half of the steaming dish, so that it covers all the holes. Put the rest of the vegetables on top of the mint and allow to steam until they are tender. Serve with Nutty Garlic and Ginger Sauce (see recipe).

Sweet and Sour Stir-Fry

1 cup cauliflower broken into flowerets
1 cup carrots, diced
1 onion, sliced
1 zucchini, sliced
1 cup green beans, halved
½ tspn basil
salt & pepper to taste

1 capsicum red, sliced
2 cloves garlic, chopped
4 eschallot, chopped
3 tbsps tamari
120 g mushrooms, sliced

Sauce
2 tspn ginger, grated
4 tbsps honey
6 tbsps vinegar
3 tbsps tamari
1/4 cup tomato paste

Mix together the sauce ingredients and leave aside. Stir-fry the onion, garlic and ginger in the tamari until the onions are translucent. Add carrots, capsicum and beans first and allow to cook for 2-3 min.

Mix in the rest of the ingredients turn down the heat and cook until the vegetables are tender but crisp, then cover and add the sauce. Stir together for a few more min. before serving. You may also add fish, chicken or tofu as there is no other protein, starch or fatty acid.

Hot Curried Vegetables

Curry

2 cups water
1 tspn tumeric
1 tspn coriander, ground

2 cloves garlic, crushed
¾ tspn chilli powder
1 tspn ginger, grated

Vegetables

1 cup green beans, halved
1 zucchini, strips
1 capsicum red, sliced
½ cup eschallots, thinly sliced
1 cup cauliflower flowerets steamed & pureed

1 carrot, cut into strips
1 stick celery, diced
6 mushrooms, sliced
1 tin tomatoes & juice

Bring water and spices to boil then turn down heat. Add vegetables, except tomatoes and eschallot, and simmer until just tender before adding the tomatoes and eschallots. Thicken with the cauliflower.As this dish contains no proteins, starches or fatty acids, it is quite an excellent accompaniment for fish or chicken lightly grilled or fried in 1-2 tbsps lemon juice.

Ratatouille

1 cup carrots, sliced
1 onion, sliced
2 cloves garlic, chopped
120 g mushrooms, sliced
4 eschallot, chopped
1 cup cauliflower broken into flowerets

1 zucchini, sliced
1 capsicum red, diced
1 cup eggplant, diced
½ tspn basil
salt & pepper to taste

Blanch carrots and cauliflower in boiling water for 3 min. then drain and pour cold water over them to prevent them cooking in their own heat. Combine with the rest of the ingredients in a saucepan with 2 tbsps water and stir over medium heat for 2-3 min. Cover and cook for 3 min. Serve with baked potatoes, fish or chicken.

Vegetable Shepherd's Pie

Vegetables
2 medium carrots, sliced
1 onion, cut in rings
150 g cauliflower flowerets
1 cup green beans, chopped

1 medium zucchini, sliced
6 mushrooms, sliced
150 g broccoli flowerets

Gravy
1 onion, finely chopped
2 cups water
½ cup parsley
1 cup cauliflower, steamed
mashed potato

2 cloves garlic crushed
1 tbsp tomato paste
1 tspn fenugreek
salt & pepper to taste

Steam 3 potatoes and mash with a small amount of salt and pepper. Sauté onion in 1-2 tbsps water then add all other gravy ingredients and simmer for 5 min. Place in blender and puree.

Put rest of vegetables into casserole dish and spoon over the gravy. Top with mashed potato then place onion rings on top and bake at 230° C until the potato is golden brown.

A green garden salad is all this dish requires.

Zucchini Creole

1 capsicum, red, sliced
4 medium zucchini, sliced

1 onion, sliced
1 tspn basil

1 can tomatoes (no salt or sugar)   salt & pepper to taste

Sauté capsicum and onion in a little of the tomato juice for 3 min., then add all the other ingredients. Cover and simmer for 10 min. over low heat. This is another vegetable dish which is an excellent accompaniment for a fish or chicken dish.

Zucchini Iskaan

1 cup steamed, pureed cauliflower
4 medium zucchini   100 g almond meal
2 onions, chopped   2 carrots, diced
1 stick celery, diced   1 capsicum red, diced
1 tspn tarragon   1 tspn dill
3 cloves garlic   1 tspn lemon juice
1 tspn hot paprika   2 bay leaves
salt & pepper to taste   ½ cup water

Sauté the onions and garlic in 1-2 tbsps tamari until translucent then add the carrots, celery, capsicum, salt and pepper, tarragon, dill and bay leaves and simmer until the vegetables are tender. Blend the almond meal with the water and zucchini pulp. Stir the lemon, cauliflower and almond meal-zucchini into the vegetables. Spoon the filling into the zucchini skins and pack them into a baking pan with 1-2 tbsps water in the bottom. Cover tightly and bake at 150ºC for 30 min. Top with chopped herbs before serving.

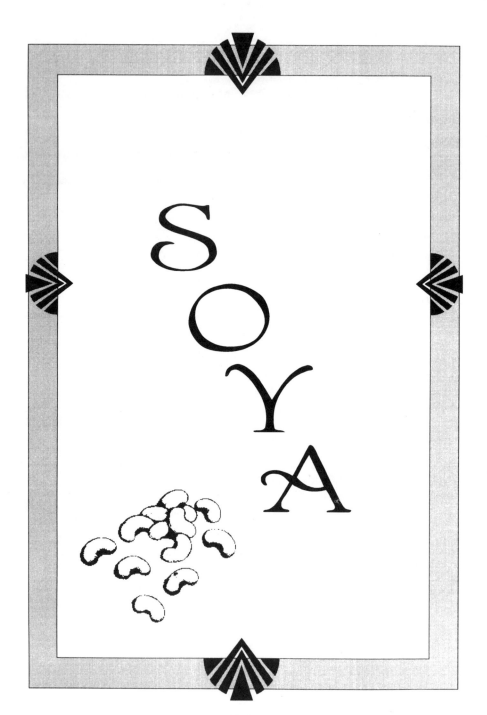

SOYA

Soya products derived from the wonderful soya bean are a nutritious and healthy alternative to meat and dairy products. They are full of protein, fat, carbohydrates, iron, isoflavones (phytoestrogens which help regulate female hormonal balance), minerals and vitamins. The benefit of soy products is that these nutrients are readily available compared to the more conventional sources.

Soy products include tofu, tempeh, hatcho miso, tamari, shoyu, soymilk and the beans themselves.

Being such a concentrated food it is important that soy products are treated as an 'eat alone' food, except for tamari, miso and shoyu which are fermented products and are therefore more readily digestible.

DIPS AND MARINADES

Dill Tofu

250 g tofu, mashed
1 tbsp fresh dill, chopped
3-4 gherkins, pickled in brine

2 tspns honey
1 tbsp lemon juice

Purée all ingredients until smooth. Chill and serve with vegetable fingers.

Tempeh Pâté

½ block tempeh
2 tbsps lime or lemon juice

1 tbsp laos
2 tbsps ketchap manis

Dice tempeh finely and dry-fry until golden brown (may also be steamed or parboiled). Place all ingredients together and pound purée or process. Add 1-2 roasted chillies and 2 cloves roasted garlic for a fiery version. Serve with slices or wedges of raw carrots for dipping.

For another version (prepare as above)

2 tbsps mustard (hot or mild)
½ block tempeh
3 tbsps hatcho miso (no added rice, etc.)
2 tbsps fresh coriander finely chopped

This paté can also be used to make stuffed mushrooms by steaming even-sized large mushrooms for 5 min. and then filling with the paté.

Pink Tofu Dip

1 eschallot, finely chopped
250 g tofu, mashed
1 medium beetroot cooked, sliced and marinated
in vinegar then drained

Purée all ingredients until smooth. Chill and serve with vegetable fingers. Alternatively make into patties and dry-fry.

Tempeh Dip

1 block tempeh
3 large tomatoes, peeled & seeded
1 tbsp coriander, roughly chopped
1 tbsp basil roughly chopped
1 tspn fresh thyme, chopped

2 tbsps miso
1 onion, finely chopped
4 tbsps vinegar
2 cloves garlic, crushed
lots fresh black pepper

2 tspns mustard powder
3 fresh red chillies or 2-3 tspns prepared chilli

Put all the ingredients except tempeh and herbs in a saucepan and simmer for 1 hour. Add herbs. Slice through tempeh to get long strips and dry-fry in some tamari. Dip with sauce.

Asian-Style Tempeh Dip

½ block of tempeh
2 small brown onions
4 medium tomatoes, well ripened

2 cloves garlic, unpeeled
4 green chillies seeded
salt to taste

The tempeh is dry-fried until crisp. Bake or grill the garlic, onions and chillies until soft (prick to avoid explosions). Also grill tomatoes until soft and the skin can be removed. Purée all ingredients and use as a side dish with vegetables.

Tomato Tofu Dip

1 tspn ginger finely grated
salt & pepper to taste
2 medium ripe tomatoes skinned & seeded

1 tbsp vinegar
250g tofu mashed

Mix cider vinegar and ginger and leave for 5 min. Pound purée or process all ingredients until smooth.

Teriyaki

1 tbsp ginger, finely grated
1 tbsp garlic, crushed
1 cup hot water

6 tbsps dark miso
1 tbsp honey

Mix all ingredients thoroughly and heat slowly until almost boiling then cool. Best if prepared a week in advance. Use on fresh tofu or grilled seafood.

Variations:
Hot – add 1 tspn hot chilli
Asian – 3 tbsps saké
Szechwan – 1 tspn ground red Szechwan pepper
Sweet & sour – 2 tbsps vinegar & 2 tbsps honey

Soy Mayonnaise

½ cup soy milk (one free of sugars, oils etc.)
2 tbsps vinegar
¼ tspn paprika   ½ tspn crushed garlic
1 cup soy oil   ¼ tspn sea salt

In this mayonnaise you are mixing the milk and oil because they are both soy products. Blend all ingredients together except the oil. Slowly add oil until the mixture reaches a creamy consistency.

MAINS

Miso Soup with Tofu

20 cm wakame seaweed   1 bay leaf
1 medium carrot, diced   250 g diced tofu
1 medium onion, thinly sliced   miso to taste
1 tspn ginger, finely grated   2 lt water
½ medium mustard or Chinese cabbage thinly sliced

Add bay leaf and carrot to cold water and bring to boil, then add onion and wakame. Simmer 10 min. covered, bring to gentle boil again and add tofu and greens. Allow to reboil, simmer covered for 5 min. Add ginger. Take a cup of broth and dissolve about 2 tbsps miso using a wooden spoon. Return to soup and simmer for 5 min. Can be refrigerated and heated, even for breakfast.

Stuffed Tofu

500 g block tofu, cut into 1 cm thick slices
250 g vegetables, boiled, mashed and drained well
½ cup basil leaves, finely chopped
1 tbsp lime juice
1 seeded chilli
1 clove garlic
2 tbsps tamari

Begin by toasting garlic and chilli by inserting a skewer and grilling over a flame. The skin should blacken then pound in a mortar and pestle (can also chop very finely). Mix with the vegetable mash, basil and lime juice.

To prepare the tofu brush both sides of the slices lightly with the tamari and dry-fry in a non-stick pan until both sides are well cooked. Remove from pan and allow to cool.

When cooled make a slit in the tofu, along top, and place 1 tbsp of the mash in each slice. Serve garnished with freshly grated carrot and lemon.

Cream of Mushroom

1 kg field mushrooms, evenly chopped
5 cloves garlic, roughly chopped
1 tspn basil dried

2 bay leaves
1 tspn sea salt
3 tbsps miso

200 g tofu, cubed   lime juice, 1 tbsp
5 cups vegetable stock, or use a vegetable bouillon cube

Dry fry garlic and bay leaf briefly then add mushrooms and cook
until mushrooms are 'sweating'. Add salt, cover and simmer rapidly
for 15 min., stirring occasionally. Add stock and basil then rapidly
return to boil. Simmer for 5 min. then use some of the juice to
dissolve the miso and tofu to make a creamy sauce, return to
soup, and purée mushrooms if you like before serving.

Marinated Grilled Tofu

Marinade
½ cup tamari   1 tspn garlic
salt & pepper to taste   2 tspns cumin
2 tspns paprika   2 tspns onion powder

Slice tofu into rectangles, pat dry and place in marinade for half
an hour to 1 hour. Grill on hot plate or non-stick pan until brown.

Optional miso sauce
2 tbsps miso   1 tspn garlic, crushed
1 tspn ginger   2 tspns honey
1 tbsp vinegar   3 tbsps water

Mix well and place in saucepan. Simmer over low heat for 10 min.

Greens and Miso

1 cup tofu mashed   1½ lt water
1 stick kombu seaweed   2 medium bok choy
1 tspn ginger, grated   3-4 tbsps miso

Bring water and kombu to boil. Remove kombu and add greens. Over high heat bring to boil again then simmer with lid on for 5 min. Dissolve miso in one cup of stock with ginger and return to soup. Add tofu, stir well and simmer for a further 5 min.

Cauliflower Tofu

1 small or ½ large cauliflower   juice of ½ lemon

Sauce
450 g tofu
4 tbsps miso, dissolved in hot water
1 cup soy milk (without any fillers, oils etc.)

Blanche cauliflower by plunging it into salted boiling water for 2-3 min. depending on size then drain. Arrange in baking tray and pour on lemon juice. Purée sauce ingredients and pour over cauliflower. Bake at 280°C for 30 min. or until it firms and gets browned.

Tofu Cottage Cheese

750 g tofu 1 tspn tamari   1 tspn dill, finely chopped
1 tspn vinegar or lemon/lime juice   1 tbsp soy oil

Mash tofu with the other ingredients then chill before serving

Tofu and Tempeh Kebabs

1 block tofu, cut into cubes
1 block tempeh, cut into cubes
2 onions in quarters, layers separated
1 each red and yellow capsicums cut into squares

Marinade
½ cup tamari
1 tbsp ginger, finely grated
2 tbsps tomato paste
1 tbsp coriander, ground
½ cup water

1 tbsp garlic, crushed
1 tbsp honey
2 tbsps vinegar
ground pepper, to taste

Arrange tofu and tempeh on skewer, alternating with onion and capsicum.

Bring the marinade slowly up to high heat and pour over skewers in flat dish. Marinate for 1 hour and grill until well browned, turning occasionally.

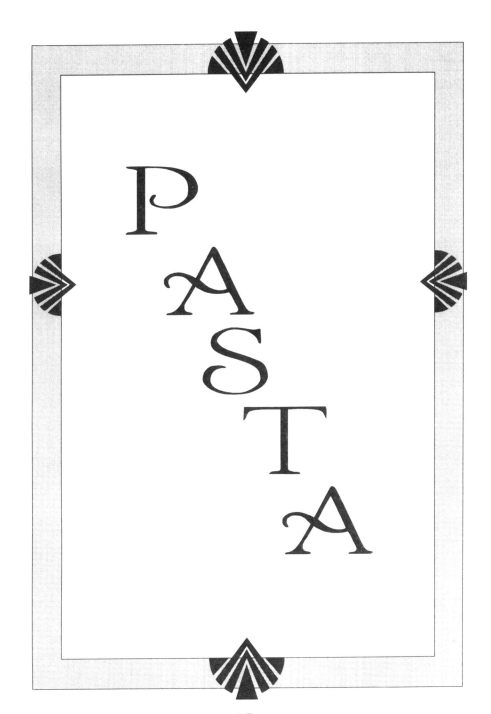

PASTA

Lasagne

1 packet corn or wholemeal lasagne sheets
1 onion, thinly sliced rings
1-2 large zucchinis, sliced

Sauce
8-10 egg tomatoes roughly chopped
200 g beans, topped & tailed, in 1 cm pieces
3 tbsps mixed fresh herbs
1 carrot finely grated
¼ head cauliflower flowerets   2 cups water
2-3 tbsps tomato paste   2 tspns hot paprika
1 tub low fat ricotta cheese   salt & pepper to taste
2 tbsps sour light cream   3-4 cloves garlic, crushed

Sauté onions until translucent then put to side. Put sauce ingredients in pot and bring to the boil and simmer. While simmering prepare lasagne sheets (follow packet instructions).

Layer zucchini on bottom of dish, spoon over sauce and cheese mix. Put on lasagne sheets. Repeat zucchini, sauce and lasagne until you get to the top then finish with the sauce mix. Cover and cook in pre heated oven at 180°C for 30-40 min.

Pasta with Roasted Peppers and Wild Mushrooms

250 g pasta (corn, wholemeal, buckwheat or other)
1 red capsicum
1 yellow capsicum
1 small onion, finely chopped
salt & pepper to taste
60 g wild mushrooms, wiped clean and torn into pieces

90 g chestnut mushrooms, wiped clean & quartered
2-4 tspns whole grain mustard (sour light cream (optional)

Preheat grill to hot and place the peppers under it to blacken the skins. Turn regularly until all skin is blackened then remove and place into plastic bag to cool. Remove skin, de-seed and slice. Cook pasta, drain, reserving 2-3 tbsps liquid, salt and pepper to taste and keep warm.

While pasta is cooking slowly dry fry the onion until soft, add peppers and cook for a few more min. until soft. Cook gently, add reserved liquid covered for 4 min., stir in mustard and cream if using. Pour the sauce over the pasta and mix in.

Mushroom Pasta

2 cups fresh tomatoes, skinned and pureed
½ kg fresh mushrooms, sliced
½ cup onion, roughly chopped
1 tspn oregano
cooked pasta of choice, kept warm
1 bay leaf
salt & pepper to taste

Add all the ingredients together, except the mushrooms and pasta, bring to boil then simmer for 15 min. over a reduced heat. Add mushrooms to tomato puree, season with salt & pepper and spoon over pasta.

Pasta Salad with Tomatoes and Beans

In this salad we mix the corn pasta (starch) and corn oil because they are the same food in a different form. Note though that the oil is not heated but added cold with dressing.

500 g corn pasta shapes	2 tbsps vinegar
1 tspn mustard	¼ cup corn oil
½ tspn honey	2 tbsps water
1 clove garlic, finely chopped	2 tspns salt
salt & pepper to taste	

2 tspns tarragon, freshly chopped or ½ tspn dried
1 bunch rocket, washed and stems removed
1 punnet cherry tomatoes, red or yellow

In a large bowl whisk together the vinegar, mustard, water, salt, honey, tarragon, garlic and pepper. Slowly add the oil in a stream, whisking all the time until the dressing becomes emulsified.

In a large saucepan of boiling salted water cook the pasta for 8-10 min. then drain and rinse well. Use a serving bowl to toss the pasta with the dressing, tomatoes and finely shredded rocket.

Vegetable Pasta

375 g corn shell pasta	1 zucchini thinly sliced
4 golden squash quartered	1 tspn marjoram
½ red capsicum, roughly chopped	1 tspn ground paprika
100 g mushrooms, thinly sliced	2 tspns basil
½ tspn black peppercorns, cracked	
3 tomatoes, peeled & roughly chopped	
3 baby eggplants, see instructions	

Cook pasta in hot salted boiling water until done to your liking. Drain and keep hot. Dry fry eggplant, capsicum, squash and zucchini for 3-4 min. Add mushrooms and cook for a further few min. Add tomatoes and remaining spices, toss together, cover and simmer for 5 min. until vegetables are tender. Finally, add pasta, toss together and serve with a lovely salad.

Broccoli and Mushroom Pasta

wholemeal or corn noodles
1 tspn miso, dissolved in hot water
100 g fresh basil, chopped
1 large bunch broccoli, in flowerets
250 g field mushrooms, sliced
3 tbsps sour light cream (if desired)

1 lemon, juice
1 onion, sliced
2 cloves garlic, crushed
150 g snow peas

Cook garlic and onion in the lemon juice, miso and a little water until onions are soft. Add the mushrooms, broccoli and basil and cook until tender. Add the snow peas at the last moment before spooning the mixture over the cooked noodles.

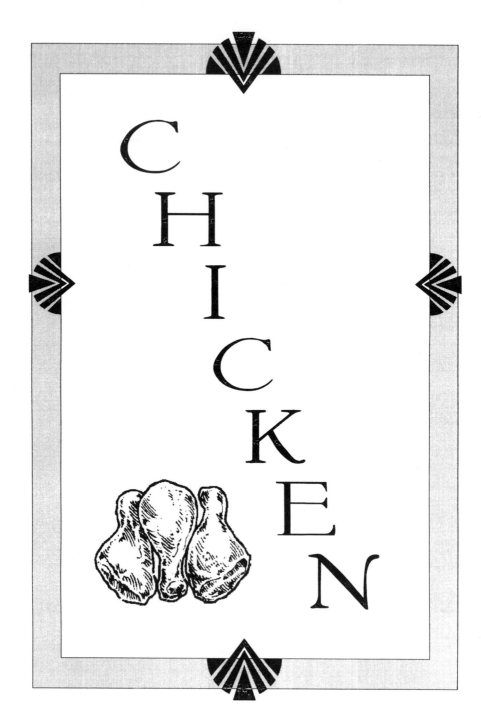

CHICKEN

Brandy and Mushroom Chicken

1 kg chicken tender loins
½ cup hot water
½ tspn bitters
2 tspns cumin
200 g mushrooms roughly chopped

¼ cup brandy
3 tspns paprika
salt & pepper to taste
juice of ½ lemon

Heat non-stick fry pan over medium heat until hot then add chicken. Sauté until lightly cooked then add lemon to stop it burning (lower heat if necessary). While the chicken is cooking combine the remaining ingredients and puree, using either a hand blender or a food processor. When the chicken is cooked, turn down the heat to low then add the puree. Cover and allow to simmer until the sauce is heated. Serve with fresh vegetables or salad.

Thai Style Grilled Chicken

1 kg chicken breasts
1 fresh chilli finely chopped
¼ cup coriander or parsley
1 red capsicum, thinly sliced
¼ cup lemon grass tea, tea bag or fresh if available

½ cup lime or lemon juice
2 cloves garlic, crushed
1 onion, thinly sliced

Make 3 diagonal slashes in each chicken half-breast. Combine salt, chilli, garlic, coriander, lemon grass tea and half the lime juice. Pour over chicken and allow to marinate in the refrigerator for several hours or overnight, turning once or twice.

Cook the chicken under a medium grill and baste often with the marinade. On a serving platter combine the onion and capsicum with the remaining lime juice, arrange the chicken on the platter and garnish with herbs.

Herb-filled Chicken Breast

4 skinless chicken breasts, open by slicing along the width
½ head broccoli & ½ head cauliflower, in medium florets
1 red capsicum, sliced
4 medium tomatoes, halved
4 yellow squash, cubed

Stuffing
½ cup mixed herbs   1 tbsp tamari
1 medium onion, finely chopped   2 cloves garlic, crushed

Marinade
2 tbsps tomato paste   1 cup lemon grass tea
1 tbsp honeysalt & pepper to taste

Preheat oven to 180°C. Dry-fry the stuffing ingredients, place on one half of the breast fillet then fold over the other half to close the pocket. The two halves may be held together by either using toothpicks or a needle and thread.

Arrange cut vegetables on the bottom of a casserole dish and place the chicken on top. Mix together the marinade and pour over the chicken and vegetables. Cover dish and place in oven. Cook for 30-40 min., remembering to baste the chicken every 15 min.

Spicy Indian Chicken

Marinated in a spicy paste for 24 hours then served with a heavily spiced sauce this is the dish for the adventurous taste buds. May also be done with fish.

1 kg skinless chicken breast fillets

Marinade

150 ml white wine

1 onion, roughly chopped

1 tspn ground cumin

2 tspns yellow mustard powder

2.5 cm fresh ginger root, peeled and roughly chopped

1 green chilli pepper, seeded and roughly chopped

2 cloves garlic, crushed

1 tspn ground coriander

1 tspn ground cinnamon

Sauce

2 eschallot, finely chopped

2 tsps black mustard seeds

½ tspn ground coriander

150-250 ml wine, to taste

juice of ½ a lime

½ tspn ground cumin

½ tspn ground turmeric

1 tbsp tomato paste

1 small green chilli pepper,

250 g peeled and chopped tomatoes seeded & finely chopped

2 tbsps finely chopped fresh coriander

Place all the marinade ingredients in a food processor and purée until smooth. Using a sharp knife make several sharp cuts in the chicken to aid the marinating process. Place in large dish and pour in the marinade, rubbing it in. Cover with film and refrigerate for 24 hours, turning and basting at least twice a day.

Remove chicken from fridge 1 hour before cooking and preheat the oven to 180°C. Place the chicken with the marinade in a pan, cover and roast for about 20 min. Remove chicken to a warmed dish and reserve the juices. To make the sauce slowly, dry-fry the eschallots until soft. Add the mustard seeds, chilli pepper, garlic and ginger, and fry for a further 2 min. Stir in the turmeric, cumin and coriander then add the tomatoes, tomato purée, white wine and any reserved juices. Cook over a low heat until slightly reduced, then stir in the lime juice and fresh coriander. You may also add 2 tbsps sour light cream. Pour sauce over chicken and serve.

Chicken Yakatori

400 g chicken, any part cut into thin strips
½ cup tamari
¼ cup honey
1 clove garlic, crushed
½ tspn ground ginger
bamboo skewers, ½ size (soaked to prevent burning)

Place chicken in bowl, mix in the tamari, honey, garlic and ginger. Cover, place in the refrigerator and allow to marinate for several hours or overnight if possible. Thread one or two strips onto the skewers using a weaving motion. Brush with marinade. Heat barbecue to high and cook for 1-2 min. on each side. Serve hot as finger food.

Red Chicken Salad

500 g chicken fillets   1 onion, thinly sliced
1 tbsp lemon juice   1 red capsicum, sliced
½ small red cabbage, finely shredded

Dressing (mix together in screw top jar and mix well)
2 tbsps coarse grained mustard
2 tbsps tamari   ½ tbsp honey
salt & pepper to taste   2 tbsps vinegar

Grill or dry-fry chicken until done then remove and drain on paper towelling. When cool cut into cubes or thin slices. Combine the remaining ingredients with the chicken and toss with the dressing just before serving.

Chicken Wings in a Glazed Lemon Sauce

20 chicken wings
¼ tspn grated lemon rind
¼ cup lemon/lime juice
1 clove garlic, crushed
4 spring onions cut into thin diagonal pieces

salt & pepper to taste
½ cup chicken stock
1 tbsp tamari
1 tbsp honey

Remove the end tip of the chicken wings (use them to make the chicken stock). Place chicken wings in a dry frying pan, season and cook over a medium heat until lightly coloured. If pan is not large enough, do in two batches and transfer to wide shallow saucepan.

Pour the stock into the pan used to cook the wings and add the lemon rind, lemon, tamari, garlic and honey and bring to boil. Pour over the wings, cover and cook for 30 min. or until they are tender. Scatter the wings with the spring onions before serving.

Barbecue Chicken with Lemon Pepper and Rosemary

8 pieces of chicken
1 punnet of cherry tomatoes
1 tbsp finely chopped parsley
4 sprigs rosemary, bruised or ½ tbsp dried rosemary
1 tbsp lemon pepper
(check it contains no fillers, starch, flour, etc.)

4 cloves garlic, crushed
3 lemons, thinly sliced

Marinate the chicken with lemon, garlic, lemon pepper, rosemary for 4 hours or overnight in the refrigerator, turning occasionally. Pat chicken dry with paper towel and barbecue until cooked – 10-12 min. approximately. Add tomatoes and grill quickly. Serve together with the parsley scattered on top.

Creamy Mustard Chicken

A special treat for those special moments.

4 chicken breasts fillets
100 ml sour light cream
2 tbsps whole grain mustard
2-3 tbsps fresh herbs, finely chopped
100 ml chicken or vegetable stock or use 3 tbsps tamari, 1 tbsp honey, stock cube and water

Put chicken in stock and bring to boil. Cover and cook for 10-15 min. Remove and keep chicken warm. Add mustard and cream boil until reduced and thickened. Return chicken and season while heating.

Honeyed Chicken

1 chicken, skinned & free range
3 tbsps honey
1 tspn mustard powder
1 tbsp tamari
salt & pepper to taste

Steam chicken (either whole or in pieces depending on the equipment available). While it is steaming combine other ingredients in small bowl. When the chicken is ready, not over-cooked so it falls apart, spread the mixture over it and brown in oven at moderate heat for 10-15 min. If the chicken is whole, turn over when top is browned. If in pieces you may brown only one or both sides as desired.

Herb Chicken

2-4 chicken breast fillets
salt & pepper to taste
1 medium onion, chopped finely
juice 1 lime and lemon (about ½ cup)
¼ tbsp hot or sweet paprika
1 cup lemon grass tea, fresh if available
1 tbsp honey dissolved in 2-3 tbsps hot water
1 cup fresh herbs – coriander, basil oregano, sage, garlic chives (to taste)

2 tbsps tamari
2 cloves garlic, crushed
½ tspn ginger powder

Combine all ingredients together in a dish and make sure the chicken is well coated. Cover and marinate as long as possible, preferably overnight. The chicken can either be dry-fried, grilled or baked in the oven with a choice of vegetables in a covered dish. Keep the marinade separate and baste the chicken often to avoid it drying out.

This recipe can also be used to prepare stuffed chicken breasts. With this variation the onion and garlic are sautéed lightly then combined with the herbs and this is used to stuff the fillets. Use toothpicks to hold together the chicken so that it keeps the stuffing in. Marinate, as above, or use the other ingredients as a basting mix. Cook as above.

Herbed Roast Chicken

Use the same ingredients as Herb Chicken to prepare the whole chicken for roasting. Skin the chicken and remove all the excess fat. Use the herb stuffing to fill cuts which have been made in the breast, thighs, drumsticks and neck area of chicken.

Baste the chicken with the marinade and especially in the

cuts as this will soak into the flesh. Sit the chicken on a stainless steel wire tray in the dish to allow any fat to run off (discard this liquid, or freeze then remove the fat to use as stock).

Cover, either with dish lid if you have one or use foil, to stop the chicken drying out. Cook at 180°C for about 2 hours or until done. Baste with the marinade every 20 min. to keep moist. When it is cooked take off the foil, baste and leave for 5-10 min. to brown. Turn chicken over and brown the other side as well.

Lemon Chicken with Zucchini and Cherry Tomatoes

1 size 15 free range chicken (skinned and cut into pieces)

Marinade
3 spring onions, finely chopped
juice of 2 lemons
1 tspn finely chopped thyme leaves
1 clove garlic, crushed

Sauce
1 punnet cherry tomatoes
3 zucchini chopped
2 tbsps freshly chopped parsley

juice of 1 lemon
1 tbsp sour light cream
1 tspn grated lemon rind

Remove skin and any excess fat from chicken. Mix marinade ingredients in a small bowl. Place chicken pieces in a shallow dish and pour over marinade. Cover and refrigerate for two hours.

To make sauce place zucchini in a pot and cook until soft. Slice cherry tomatoes in half and add to zucchini with the other ingredients for a few min. Season with salt and pepper to taste. Grill or barbecue chicken until cooked then arrange on plate and pile around zucchini and tomato mixture.

Satay Chicken

2 skinned chicken thigh fillets   1 tspn curry powder
2 tspn honey   2 tbsps tamari
2 tbsps sour light cream
½ cup water
1 chicken stock cube (ensure it is free of fillers)
½ tspn sambal oelek (chilli sauce – ensure it is free of fillers or you may use the chilli paste described earlier)

Mix all the ingredients, except the water, together in a bowl, add the chicken pieces and allow to marinate for 20-30 min. Remove the chicken from the marinade and grill or dry fry. Mix the remaining marinade with the water, heat lightly and use as a sauce.

Tandoori Chicken

12 skinless chicken pieces   1 tspn garlic powder
1 tspn ground ginger   1 tbsp ground paprika
1 tspn garam masala   2 tspn ground turmeric
juice of 1 lemon   1 onion, sliced
garnish – 2 limes, cut in wedges

Combine lemon juice and spices to make the tandoori mix. Rub the mixture into the chicken, coating thoroughly. Arrange in a single layer in a flat baking dish. Cover and leave in the refrigerator for 12 - 24 hours.

Cover tray with foil and cook in a hot oven (200ºC) for 20 min. Reduce heat to moderate (180ºC) and bake for a further 30 min. (Take off foil for the last 10-15 min. to brown).

Arrange on a platter and garnish with lime wedges and onion slices.

Slow-cooked Eggs

6 large eggs
Outer skins from 3 to 4 onions
1 tbsp olive oil

You will need a deep saucepan with a lid. Wrap the onion skins around the eggs and place the eggs in a deep saucepan; the eggs should fit somewhat snugly in the pan so that they don't rattle around and crack when cooking.

Add enough cold water to cover the eggs by 25-50 ml. Pour in the olive oil, which helps reduce the amount of water that evaporates during cooking. Cover the saucepan, and cook over the lowest possible heat for at least 6 hours, or as long as overnight, checking occasionally to make sure there is sufficient water.

Serve warm or at room temperature. They will keep for several weeks in the refrigerator, but are best eaten, unrefrigerated within a day of cooking.

Chicken Ratatouille

2 chicken breasts, skinned & boned, cut into bite sized pieces
1 cup carrots
1 cup cauliflower, in flowerets   1 onion, sliced
1 capsicum red, diced   1 zucchini, sliced
2 cloves garlic, chopped   120 g mushrooms, sliced
1 cup eggplant, diced   4 eschallots, chopped
½ tspn basil   2 tspn paprika
salt & pepper to taste   1 tspn thyme
1 tbsp parsley, chopped
spicy tomato sauce (see recipe)

Sprinkle chicken pieces with pepper and paprika then gently brown in non-stick pan. When cooked remove and keep warm. Blanch carrots and cauliflower in boiling water for 3 min. then drain and pour cold water over them to prevent them cooking in their own heat.

Combine with the rest of the ingredients in a saucepan with 2 tbsps water and stir over medium heat for 2-3 min. Cover and cook for 3 min. Arrange vegetables on a hot platter with the chicken on top and then sprinkle on the parsley and serve with Spicy Tomato Sauce.

Curried Chicken

1 onion, chopped
¾ tspn chilli paste or powder
1 tspn ground coriander
250 g mushrooms
4 eschallots, sliced
2 tsps tumeric

2 cloves garlic
½ tspn ground ginger
2 cups water
2 zucchini, chopped
2 chicken breasts

Sauté onion and garlic lightly in 4 tbsps water then add tumeric, chilli, ginger and coriander. Cook for 2 min., add chicken pieces and sauté for 2 min. before adding the rest of the water. Cover and simmer until chicken is tender then add the remainder of the vegetables and cook for a further 5 min.
Try this combination with a Green Bean Salad.

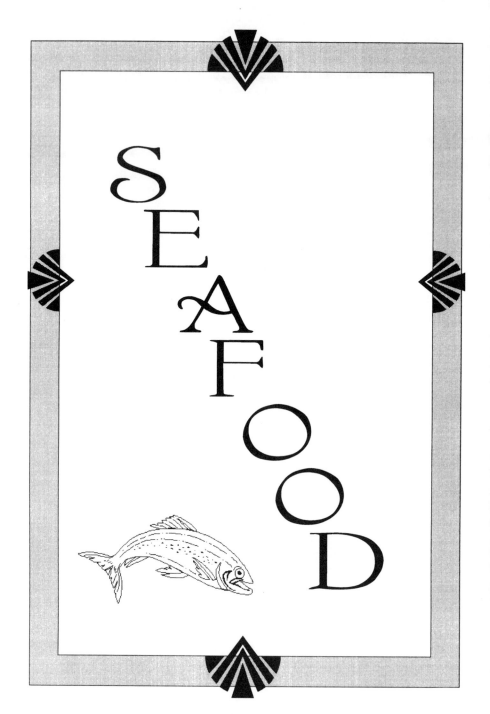

SEAFOOD

Chilli Prawns

750 g green prawns, shelled and de-veined
1 cup tomato sauce

1 tbsp honey   6 eschallots, chopped
2 tspns crushed garlic   2 tspns crushed ginger
1 tbsp tamari   2 tspns chilli (see recipe)

Combine tomato sauce with honey. Add the garlic, ginger and chilli to the wok and cook over a medium heat until lightly browned. Add the tomato mixture and eschallots and simmer for 2-3 min. before adding the prawns. Simmer until just cooked and serve with a green garden salad or vegetables.

Gingered Fish

4 thick fish fillets   2 tspns crushed ginger
6 eschallots, finely chopped   2 tbsps tamari
2 tbsps parsley, chopped   salt & pepper to taste
125 g mushrooms, thinly sliced

Place fish in centre of a piece of aluminium foil large enough to enclose the fish completely. Sprinkle with some of the parsley, eschallots, salt and pepper and ginger. Repeat with the other pieces of fish. Fold up foil like parcel and cook either on barbecue or in moderate oven for 10 - 15 min. until fish is tender.

Salmon Dip/Sauce

415 g salmon in brine or spring water
1/3 cup tamari
2 tbsps tomato paste   2 tspns paprika

2 tbsps curry powder

juice of ½ a lime

2 tspns seeded mustard

3 tbsps herb vinegar

1 tspn onion powder

½ cup fresh herbs (basil, coriander, parsley) chop finely

mixed vegetables for dipping sticks.

To make the dip into a thinner sauce add 4 to 6 medium tomatoes skinned and pureed or alternately use a can of tomatoes.

Blend all ingredients together then heat over a medium flame until all the ingredients are heated thoroughly. As a dip use vegetables of your choice and cut them into finger size servings. As a sauce pour over your favourite vegies and serve with a fresh garden salad.

Lemon Grass Fish

4 white fish fillets

½ cup lemon grass tea

2 tspns crushed garlic

1 tbsp lime or lemon juice

3 tspns finely grated ginger

3 tspns chilli paste

1 tspn green peppercorns, chopped

Combine all marinade ingredients and mix up thoroughly. Place fish in flat dish, cover with marinade and allow to stand for 15-30 min. Barbecue, grill or pan fry, turning only once and brushing with marinade. Serve with mixed lettuce salad.

Sardines with Lemon and Herbs

500 g fresh sardines

juice of 1 lemon

1 tspn chopped fresh oregano

2 tspns each of fresh thyme & parsley, finely chopped

Rub off the scales from the sardines with a cloth or soft paper. Rinse and dry the fish. Cut the heads off by cutting from the backbone. Open out the fish enough to lift out the guts and backbone, cutting it off with scissors close to the tail but leaving the tail on. Rinse and dry the fish and reform to original shape.

Place sardines in a shallow dish. Mix together the lemon juice and half the herbs and pour the mixture over the fish. Marinate for about 10 min., turning them over once or twice.

Cook the sardines either on a grill, non-stick pan or barbecue until they are golden brown and serve hot with salad or vegetables.

Dill-cured Salmon

750g fresh salmon, halved along backbone and all bones removed. If not whole fish then 2 large slices
3 tbsps coarse sea salt
1 large bunch dill
1 tbsp crushed peppercorns
1 tbsp honey

If the salmon is whole scrape off the scales and pat dry with kitchen towel. Place a handful of dill on a large plate and place one half of the salmon on top, skin side down. Combine the honey, salt and peppercorns and spread over the salmon. Add another handful of dill and cover with the remaining salmon, skin side up. Cover with the remaining dill.

Cover the entire plate with film and place a plate on top, weighted with a heavy object. Place in the refrigerator for at least 48 hours but not longer than three days. Baste the salmon twice each day with the juices produced, separating the salmon halves slightly to baste inside. When ready to serve, remove the salmon from the fridge, scrape clean and pat dry. Slice thinly using a sharp knife. Serve with a mustard sauce or other condiments of your choice. If salmon is not available use fresh tuna.

Spicy Crab Claws

16-24 crab claws
4 eschallots, finely chopped
1 tspn seeded mustard
2 red chilli peppers, finely chopped
250 g tomatoes, peeled and chopped

salt & pepper to taste
1 clove garlic, crushed
300 ml fish or vegie stock

Put eschallots into pot with garlic and chilli peppers and cook over a low flame until soft but not browned. Pour in the stock add the tomatoes, stir in the mustard then season and bring to the boil. Add the crab claws, reduce the heat and simmer for a few min. Serve with wonderfully fresh salad or vegetables.

Pickled Octopus

1½ kg baby octopus
1 cup vinegar
salt & pepper to taste
½ cup honey
½ cup finely chopped herbs (basil, oregano, dill, parsley)

4 cloves garlic,
¼ tamari
½ tspn paprika
½ onion, finely chopped

To prepare the baby octopus remove the beak by prising it out with a pointed knife, then rinse and drain. Add all ingredients together in saucepan, bring to boil and then simmer until the octopus is tender, about 15 min. Place in jars and top up with the liquid remaining in the pan. Allow to cool and store in fridge.

(This recipe can also be used for any other seafood e.g. mussels, calamari, etc.)

Fish In Tomato Sauce

4 pieces of firm fish
1 tbsp parsley, chopped
1 tspn cumin powder
salt & pepper to taste

2 cloves garlic, crushed
1 tbsp basil, chopped
500 g skinned & peeled tomatoes

Place ingredients, except fish, in pan and cook for 5-10 min. then pour half of sauce into shallow dish and lay fish on top and cover with remaining sauce. Cover and cook in oven at 190°C for 15-20 min.

Fish Chowder Supreme

2-3 fish fillets, firm fleshed e.g. dory or king cut into small squares
1 red capsicum, chopped
2 eschallots, chopped
1 cup chopped green beans
150 g mushrooms
1 tbsp cumin
1 tspn each of cinnamon & mustard
½ cup coriander and parsley, chopped
salt & pepper to taste

1 onion, chopped
2 tomatoes, chopped
2 cloves garlic, chopped
1 cup water

Place mushrooms, herbs and spices in saucepan with the water to simmer. In another frypan sauté the onions and garlic until the onions are translucent then add other vegetables and cook over low heat. Puree the mushroom mixture and mix in with the ingredients in the frypan, add the fish, cover and simmer until the fish is cooked.

Stir-fry with Salmon Sauce

Sauce
415 g red salmon (in brine), save liquid
2 medium onions   2 tbsps salsa
2 cloves garlic, crushed   fresh basil
salt & pepper to taste   1 chilli fresh

Dry-fry the onion and garlic for 2 min. then add the remaining ingredients (except for the salmon which is added a few min. before serving) and simmer over low heat while you prepare the stir-fry.

Stir- fry

4 brussel sprouts, quartered   100 g beanshoots
2 eschallots, finely chopped   1 yellow zucchini, diced
1 cup shredded red cabbage   100 g oyster mushrooms

Heat some lemon juice in a wok and add the zucchini, brussel sprouts and cabbage first as these take a bit longer to cook. Cook for a few min. then add the remainder of the ingredients and continue until they are nearly ready. Add the salmon to the sauce for a few min. to heat it up then pour on top of the stir fry and serve.

Prawns with Asparagus

1 kg green prawns   1 tbsp garlic, crushed
1 red capsicum, roughly chopped   1 tbsp curry powder
2 tbsps lemon grass tea   1 tbsp ginger, crushed
2 bunches of asparagus cut in half
1 yellow capsicum, roughly chopped

Shell the prawns, leaving the tails on. Add garlic, ginger and curry to wok or frypan and cook for 1 min. in the lemon grass tea. Add half of the prawns and cook until done. Add the remaining prawns, cook and remove. Quickly stir-fry the asparagus, capsicum and spring onions until done. Return the prawns to the wok or frypan and toss until heated.

Baked Fish

fish (fillets or whole)   ½ lemon, sliced
3 tomatoes   ¼ cup lemon juice
½ stick celery, sliced
salt & pepper to taste

Place a layer of tomatoes and celery on the bottom of a casserole dish then lay the fish on top. Add the lemon juice, with half tbsps. water, before adding another layer of tomato and slices of lemon on top of the fish. Add salt & pepper to taste, cover and cook in oven at 180º C until tender.

Serve the fish on a platter surrounded by steamed vegetables, a mushroom sauce and side salad.

Fish and Vegetable Casserole

firm white fish fillets   1 onion, sliced
2 cloves garlic   1 lemon, sliced
3 tomatoes, sliced   1 capsicum red, sliced
2 tbsps parsley   juice 1 lemon

Sauté onions and garlic in 2 tbsps. water then add tomatoes, capsicum and parsley and simmer for 5 min. Place fish in casserole dish and season with salt and pepper and lemon. Cover with vegetables and bake at 200ºC for 20 min. When nearly cooked, top with the lemon slices.

A side serve of cucumber, tomato and sunflower sprouts with a light lemon dressing complements this dish superbly.

Tuna Casserole

1 can tuna in brine or spring water, drained

1 onion medium	1 capsicum, red
2 eschallot	¼ cup coriander
2 zucchinis	1 carrot grated
100 g green beans	100 g mushrooms
2 cloves garlic	¼ cup parsley
1 tspn cumin	1 tspn curry powder
4 cups water	salt & pepper

Roughly chop all the vegetables as we want a chunky appearance to this casserole. Lightly dry sauté onion, garlic and eschallots with the spices until onions become translucent. Add the tuna, with the rest of the ingredients, to a saucepan and bring contents to the boil then simmer for 20 min.

Serve with a shredded lettuce and tomato salad topped with sunflower sprouts.

Tuna Stuffed Peppers

2 capsicums red, topped and seeded

2 ½ cups celery, finely chopped	1 can tuna, drained
3 tbsps spicy tomato sauce	1 onion, chopped
½ tspn thyme	1 tbsp lemon juice

Sauté onion in a little water and add to the rest of the ingredients.

Fill the capsicum halves with the mixture and bake at 180º C for 20 min. Arrange the peppers on a lettuce leaf with some shredded white and red cabbage.

Tali Machi

¾-1 kg fish steaks
1½ tspns rock salt
1 tspn finely grated fresh ginger
½ tspn ground black pepper

2 cloves garlic, crushed
½ tspn ground turmeric
lemon juice
½ tspn chilli powder

Wash fish and dry on paper towel. Mix garlic with salt and other spices and enough lemon juice to make a paste. Rub well over both sides of the fish, cover and leave for 20 min. Dry-fry one side over a medium heat in a non-stick pan then carefully turn over and cook until done.

Spicy Steamed Mussels

1 kg mussels
½ tspn ground turmeric
2 large onions, finely chopped
4 cloves garlic, finely chopped
3 tspns ginger finely chopped
1 tbsp fresh chopped coriander leaves
3 fresh red chillies, seeded & chopped

lemon juice to taste
½ tspn salt
1 cup water
3 tspns coriander powder

Scrub and beard mussels. Fry onion, garlic and ginger then add chilli, turmeric, coriander and stir for 3-5 min. Add salt and water. Bring to boil then simmer for 5 min. Add mussels, cover and steam for 10-15 min. or until opened. Remove from heat and spoon gravy over.

Squid Sambal

500 g squid
2 onions finely chopped
½ tspn dried shrimp paste
2 cloves garlic
2 strips lemon rind
5 fresh red chillies
2 tspns honey
1-2 tspns paprika
¼ cup tamarind liquid or 1 tspn tamarind paste

Clean squid, discarding clear spine if present, and cut into rings. Put onion, garlic, shrimp paste, lemon rind and chillies into blender and puree. Dry-fry mixture until dark then add tamarind liquid, honey and paprika and stir in squid. Serve with vegetables when squid is cooked.

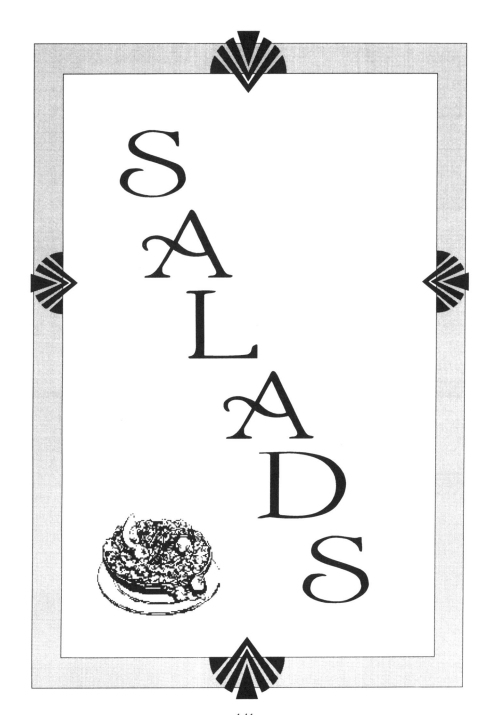

SALADS

Brown Rice and Mustard Salad

2 cups brown rice
3 tbsps basil, finely chopped
1½ tbsps lemon juice or vinegar
1 red capsicum, seeded and diced
3-4 eschallots & 3 stalks celery, thinly sliced
2 tspns mustard of choice
salt & pepper to taste

Bring 4 cups salted water to the boil in a heavy saucepan. Meanwhile, wash the rice thoroughly then sprinkle it into the boiling water so that the water remains at the boil. Boil for a few min. then cover tightly. Turn the heat to very low and cook without lifting the lid for about 40-50 min. If it is cooked at this time, uncover for a few min. to allow the steam to escape, then fluff up with a fork. Cool to room temperature.

Blend the mustard, salt, pepper, and lemon juice or vinegar together. Toss the rice with the dressing. Add the celery, spring onions and diced pepper. Toss lightly and season well with salt & pepper.

Bean Salad

½ kg green beans lightly steamed
½ cup chopped parsley and mint, juice of 1 lemon
dash of tamari
½ onion finely chopped (soaked in water for ½ hour to get the strong odour out. Drain well.)

Mix all ingredients together and serve with main meal. Excellent summer entree.

Salmon Salad

415 g tin salmon in brine (save brine for dressing)

½ medium cucumber chopped

4 lettuce leaves roughly sliced

1 yellow squash thinly sliced

1 red capsicum thinly sliced

cup red cabbage finely shredded

2 tomatoes, chopped

handful sprouts

1 carrot, finely shredded

5-6 mushrooms chopped

Dressing

juice from tinned salmon

2 tbsps tamari

pepper to taste

juice of ½ lemon

2 tbsps vinegar

Combine salad and dressing ingredients in a bowl and mix well. Serve with Gaspachio cold soup and Bean Salad for a wonderful summer lunch.

Endive Salad with Mustardy Egg Dressing

250 g tender endive leaves, washed and dried

2 hard boiled eggs, roughly chopped

Dressing

2 hard boiled egg yolks

2 tbsps tamari

2 tspns cumin

chopped herbs optional

1 tspn coarse grained mustard (see recipe)

juice of 1 lemon

2 tspns paprika

salt & pepper to taste

Prepare dressing by mashing egg yolks through a sieve into a bowl then beat together with the mustard, spices and lemon juice until smooth, adding salt and pepper to taste. Slowly add the tamari until it has a creamy consistency. Set aside. Arrange prepared endive leaves and eggs on serving plates. Drizzle over the dressing and serve.

Warm Tofu and Tomato Salad

250 g tofu, cut into small cubes
1 tbsp coriander, finely chopped
2 tspns garlic, crushed
4 tomatoes, peeled
1 tbsp ginger, finely grated

1 tbsp honey
1 tbsp chilli paste
1 onion, sliced
lettuce for serving
1 tbsp lemon grass tea

Process chilli, ginger, garlic, onion, coriander, tomato lemon grass tea and honey until it becomes a smooth paste. Cook tofu in tamari until golden brown then add paste and stir until all ingredients are heated through. Serve on a bed of lettuce and garnish with some chopped herbs.

Champignon Salad

400-500 g mushrooms, washed and sliced
½ tspn pepper, freshly ground
¼ cup parsley, finely chopped
3 cloves garlic, crushed
3 tbsps fresh lemon juice

¼ cup olive oil
1 tspn mustard
1 tspn salt

Wash, pat dry and slice mushrooms then place in a bowl. Mix salt, and pepper, garlic and mustard into lemon juice. Blend well, add olive oil and blend again. Pour over salad, let marinate one hour and adjust seasoning if necessary. Serve chilled on lettuce leaves.

Mixed Tomato Salad with Mustard Dressing

750 g selection of ripe tomatoes, i.e., cherry, roma, etc.
2 tbsps apple cider vinegar
2 tspns coarse grained mustard   salt & pepper to taste
2 tbsps fresh tarragon, chopped   1 clove garlic, crushed
6 tbsps extra virgin olive oil   1 tbsp lime juice

Cut any large tomatoes into eighths, medium sized ones into quarters and cherry tomatoes in half. Combine all the ingredients except the tarragon together and pour over tomatoes and mix well. Sprinkle with tarragon and serve.

Note: the oil used in this dish means this salad cannot be mixed with any other starch protein or fatty acid.

Mustardy Potato Salad

500 g new potatoes, washed with skins on
1 tbsp mustard of choice
2 tbsps tomato paste   1 clove garlic, crushed
1 tbsp freshly squeezed lime juice   ½ tspn tabasco sauce
2 tbsps fresh oregano, chopped   salt & pepper to taste

Place the potatoes in a saucepan of cold water, bring to the boil then simmer for 10-15 min., or until tender. While the potatoes are cooking combine all the other ingredients.

When cooked drain the potatoes, rinse under cold water and drain again transfer to a large bowl, pour over the dressing and mix well.

Artichoke Heart and Tomato Salad

4 tomatoes, cut in wedges
6-8 artichoke hearts, halved
2 tbsps apple cider vinegar
2 cloves garlic, crushed

1 tbsp tarragon
1 tbsp basil
¼ cup oil of choice
salt & pepper to taste

If necessary the artichoke hearts may be canned but make sure they have no additives. Blend the marinade ingredients and pour over the tomatoes and artichoke then chill for 20 min. Serve on a bed of greens with fish

Asparagus and Sesame Seed Salad

500 g asparagus, fresh
1 tspn honey
1 tbsp apple cider vinegar
2 tbsps sesame seeds, toasted

2 tbsps tamari
½ tspn chilli paste
1 tspn ginger, grated

Remove the ends of the asparagus and put them into the boiling water and cover until the water begins to boil again (it stops when you add the asparagus). Cook until they are tender but until crisp (about 1-2 min.) then plunge into cold water and drain well. Mix together the remainder of the ingredients and pour over the asparagus. Chill for 30 min. and top with the sesame seeds before serving. May also be served hot.

Beetroot Salad

2 boiled/steamed beetroots
3 cloves garlic (crushed)
¼ cup lemon

½ cup oil
¼ cup vinegar

Cut beetroot into pieces and place in bowl. Mix all the other ingredients well in a jar and pour over beetroot. Mix well and chill overnight before serving with a main dish.

Buckwheat Salad

green leaf salad mix
1 tomato, sliced
sunflower seed sprouts
cooked buckwheat

fresh herbs to taste
4-5 mushrooms
grated fresh beetroot

Cook buckwheat in steamer until it has expanded to nearly double its size and is soft then add to other ingredients. Garnish with dressing of your choice which contains no oil.

Broccoli and Mushroom and Tofu Salad

1 cake tofu, pressed
1 bunch broccoli, in flowerets

150 g mushrooms
3 eschallots, chopped

Marinade
6 tbsps vinegar
6 tbsps tamari
pinch cayenne

1 tbsp ginger, grated
3 cloves garlic, crushed
¼ tspn fennel seeds

To press the tofu place cake between 2 plates and weight the top down until the sides of the tofu start to bulge. Do not split. Let stand for 30 min. then remove the press and drain off water before cutting into cubes. Steam the broccoli until it just starts to turn bright green and add the mushrooms for another min. or two. Rinse with cold water to prevent further cooking and drain. Combine with the eschallots in a bowl and allow to stand.

Whisk together the marinade ingredients and pour half over the vegetables and half over the tofu in another bowl. Allow to marinate for an hour, turning the vegetables and tofu several times. Mix everything together just before serving. Goes well with a green or sprout salad.

Capsicum and Capers

4-5 capsicums red, sliced	¼ cup oil
2 tbsps vinegar	1 tbsp capers, in brine
1 onion, thinly sliced	2 cloves garlic, crushed
1 tbsp tamari	salt & pepper to taste

Fry capsicums in the tamari until they are well cooked and start to brown slightly. Place the fried peppers, onion and capers, which have been drained, in a bowl and dress them with the oil, vinegar, garlic, salt and pepper. Toss well and chill. This tangy salad may be served on some greens as a side salad or as a topping for baked fish.

Tunafish Salad

1 can tuna in brine	2 cloves garlic crushed
1 onion finely chopped	2 tbsps tomato paste
1 tspn hot paprika	juice ½ lemon
fresh ground pepper	

Side salad

cabbage, finely sliced	1 medium carrot, grated
3 tomatoes, sliced	2 tbsps vinegar
1 tbsp tamari	2 tbsps lemon
1 cucumber (continental), sliced chopped mint & parsley	

Mash Tuna with the other ingredients and serve on a chilled lettuce leaf. Mix together the side salad ingredients, except the mint and parsley, and place on plate with tuna. Sprinkle the mint & parsley over the top of the tuna and salad.

Moroccan Salad

1 cup couscous, dry
1 cup carrots, diced
1 cup green beans, cut
1/3 cup red onions, finely chopped

½ tspn salt
1 capsicum red, diced
1 cup boiling water

Marinade
¼ cup lemon juice
1 tspn salt
1 tbsp spearmint
pinch cayenne

3 tbsps lime juice
¼ tspn cinnamon
¼ cup parsley, chopped

Put the couscous and salt in a large bowl and stir in the boiling water. Cover and let sit for 10-15 min., stirring occasionally to fluff. Meanwhile, steam the carrots, beans and peppers and when tender add them to the couscous. Stir in the onion before adding the marinade ingredients, which have been mixed together, and toss. Chill at least an hour to allow the flavours to combine before serving.

Carrot and Coriander Salad

3 carrots, grated
3 cloves garlic, crushed
¼-½ bunch coriander, finely chopped

½ lemon
1 tbsp oil

Mix all ingredients together in bowl and it is ready to go.

Lemon Cabbage with Walnuts

¼ head red cabbage
1 lemon, juice
2 tspns fresh ground pepper

¼ head white cabbage
50 g walnuts, crumbled

Cut cabbage into thin slices and put into steamer, which is sitting over boiling water. Add the pepper and pour the lemon juice over the cabbage so that it runs through to the water. As the water boils the lemon will come through and flavour the cabbage. Steam until tender then put into bowl and sprinkle nuts over the top and serve with curried vegetables.

Mint and Carrot Salad

¼ cup fresh mint, chopped
3 tbsps lemon juice
1 tspn salt
½ tspn coriander seeds, ground

4 carrots, grated
3 tbsps oil
1-2 tsps honey

Mix all the ingredients together and chill at least one hour before serving.

Minted Mushrooms or Beetroots

250 g mushrooms or beetroots, thinly sliced
½ cup finely chopped mint
1 cup vinegar
2 tbsps honey
½ cup water

Combine mushrooms or beetroots with mint. Bring water, vinegar and honey to boil while continually stirring. Remove from flame and pour over mushrooms or beetroots and stir in well. Refrigerate until required.

Sweet and Sour Red Cabbage

1 onion, chopped
6 cups red cabbage, thinly sliced
1 tspn fennel seeds, whole

1 tbsp dill, fresh
1 tbsp honey
3-6 tbsps vinegar

Sauté the onions lightly then add the cabbage and continue to cook for a further 10 min. Stir in the rest of the ingredients, except the honey, and cook on low heat for a further 20 min., stirring occasionally. The cabbage sweetens as it cooks so after tasting add honey or vinegar as required. Serve with another dish which is tangy to complement the sweetness of the cabbage and onion.

Sprout Salad

2 cups sprouts
1 tspn thyme
1 tbsp tamari
½ cup parsley, chopped
juice of ½ lemon

2 cloves garlic
1 onion, chopped
1 tspn fenugreek powder
2 tbsps oil

Mix all ingredients in bowl and serve with some Minted Steamed Vegetables.

Sunflower Salad

2 cups mixed sprouts
½ cup sunflower sprouts

3 egg tomatoes
1 eschallot, sliced

2 nasturtium flowers   50 g sunflower seeds
4 radishes

Dressing
tamari, lemon juice, vinegar, salt & pepper to taste

Combine mixed sprouts, sliced tomatoes and chopped eschallots
and radishes. Lightly heat sunflower seeds with a dash of tamari.
When cooled sprinkle over salad, garnish with nasturtium flowers
and sprinkle dressing over the top.

Curried Egg Salad

4 boiled eggs (5 min. in boiling water), cooled and peeled
1 salad onion, finely chopped   2 tsps curry
fresh ground black pepper   1 tspn paprika
lettuce shredded   2 tomatoes, sliced
radishes, sliced   sunflower sprouts

Chop eggs with curry until egg is well coated. Lay on a bed of
lettuce and surround with tomato and radishes. Sprinkle with
onion and top with sunflower sprouts.

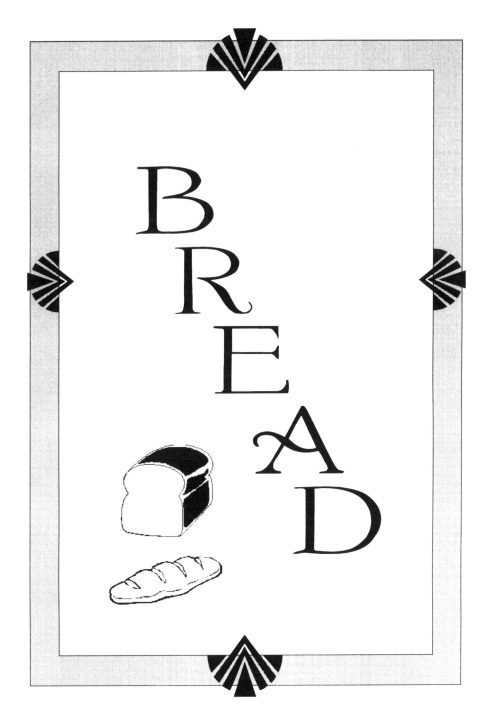

BREAD

Chapattis

2 cups atta flour (finely ground wheat flour) or sifted whole wheat flour
1 tspn salt
1 cup warm water, or more if needed

Mix together the flour and salt in a medium-sized bowl. Make a well in the centre and add the warm water. Mix, using hand or spoon, until you can gather it together into a kneadable dough (you may need to add more water or flour to get the right consistency). On a lightly floured board knead the dough for 8-10 min., cover with plastic wrap and let stand for 30 min. to 2 hours.

Divide the dough into 8 pieces and flatten with lightly floured fingers. Roll each piece out, without flipping it over, using a rolling pin to an 8 inch round. Lightly flour board as needed to prevent sticking. Cover the finished breads with plastic wrap as you finish the rest and do not stack the breads.

Heat a cast pan or non-stick pan over medium heat and when it is hot place a chapatti, top side down onto it. Cook for 10 seconds, then gently flip it over. Cook on the second side until small bubbles begin to form, about 1 min. Turn the chapatti back to the first side cook about 1 min. longer. At this stage it should start to balloon. Gently press on the bubble forcing it to expand (use a folded paper or cloth towel). Remove and wrap in tea towel to keep warm and soft. Cook the remaining breads, stacking on top of each other.

Unleavened Bread

2 cups wholemeal self raising flour
1 tspn cumin powder   1 tspn coriander powder

1 onion, finely chopped
2 tspns crushed garlic
1 cup water 1 tspn salt & pepper
1 tbsp fresh basil, finely chopped
2 tspns baking powder (6 if the flour is not self raising)

Mix all the ingredients together until you have a firm dough and bake at 180°C for 30-40 min.

Wholemeal Damper

6 cups wholemeal flour
2 tspns salt
2 cups water
1 onion, minced
1 tspn baking powder (see Appendix)
1 tbsp each of parsley, thyme and sage.

Mix the flour, salt and baking powder in bowl. Add water, onion and herbs to form a dough. Form into wide roll, place on non-stick tray and bake in a pre-heated oven at 220°C for 15-20 min.

Savoury Corn Bread

1 cup polenta
1 tspn baking powder
¼ tspn baking powder
1 cup buttermilk
1 tbsp corn oil
sprinkle paprika
1 tbsp coriander, chopped
3 cloves garlic, crushed

Combine dry ingredients in bowl, add buttermilk and mix thoroughly. Add crushed garlic and coriander and mix then add oil to batter. Very lightly oil surface of square baking tin. Pour into tin, sprinkle with paprika and cook for 20 min. at 180 °C. Serve with a lovely vegetable soup or salad.

Xichuan Pepper Bread

Xichuan peppercorn should have a strong fragrant aroma. A Chinese grocery is the best place to find these. The dough is made with both boiling water, which cooks the starches in the flour and makes a very soft dough, and cold water, which yields a stronger dough. The mix produces a soft, pliable dough, which is also elastic enough to take rolling out.

Dough

3 cups unbleached flour

1 tspn salt

½ cup plus 2 tbsps cold water

2 tspns baking powder

½ cup boiling water

Filling

1 tspn Xichuan peppercorns dry-roasted and finely ground
1 cup finely chopped eschallots (white & tender green parts) or
1 cup finely chopped garlic chives
1 cup tamari

You will need a food processor, a rolling pin and one or two heavy skillets or non-stick pans, at least 20 centimetres in diameter.

Place the flour, baking powder, and salt in a food processor and pulse to mix well. With the motor running, pour the boiling water in a thin stream through the feed tube and then add the cold water and process until the mixture forms a ball. Process for 1 min. longer, then turn the dough out onto a lightly floured surface. Knead briefly, then cover with plastic wrap and let sit for 15 min.

Divide the dough into 8 equal pieces. Working with one piece at a time, leaving the others covered, roll out the dough on a lightly floured surface to a circle 20 cm. in diameter. Spread ½ tspn of the tamari over the top of the bread, then sprinkle on ¼ tspn of the Xichuan pepper. Spread 2 tablespoons of the chopped eschallots or garlic chives evenly over the bread. Then, roll the bread as tightly as possible. Anchoring one end of the resulting tube on your work surface, coil the bread as tightly as possible and pinch the other end against the coil to make a smooth round. Flatten gently with the palm of your hand. Roll the bread out again gently with a rolling pin until it is about ¼ inch thick and 15 cm. across. (Do not worry if the odd piece of eschallot or garlic chive leaks out; you can patch any small holes in the dough.)

Place a heavy skillet over medium heat. When the skillet is hot, lower the heat to medium-low and place the first bread in the skillet. Cook for 3 min., or until the bottom is flecked with light brown spots. Turn over and cook for 3 min. or longer, or until both sides are flecked with light brown. Transfer the bread to a rack to cool slightly, then wrap in a towel to keep soft.

Meanwhile, continue rolling out and shaping the remaining breads while the first one bakes, then cook them in the same manner. If you are feeling comfortable about cooking times, heat another skillet so that you can have two breads cooking at once. Makes 8 round breads. Serve warm.

Pizza Bread Base

2 cups self raising wholemeal flour	1 cup water
2 tspns baking powder	2 tspns cumin powder
1 tspn coriander powder	1 tspn salt
1 tbsp basil, finely chopped	pinch pepper
1 onion, finely chopped	garlic to taste

Mix together and add enough water to form a firm dough. Pile on tomato paste, your pizza toppings, ricotta cheese and bake until cooked (180°C for about 20 min.).

Salt and Spice Bread

2 cups unbleached bread flour   1 cup water
1½ tspns black peppercorns   1 tspn salt
¼ cup chopped fresh coriander   2 tspns cumin seed

Place the flour in a medium bowl. Make a well in the centre, and add the water, stirring it into the flour, until a soft but not sticky dough forms. Turn out onto a lightly floured surface and knead until smooth.

Rinse out the bowl, set the dough back in the bowl, and cover with plastic wrap. Let stand for 30 min. to 1 hour. While the dough is resting, dry-roast the cumin seeds in a small heavy skillet, stirring constantly, until they just start to change colour. Transfer to a spice grinder or mortar and grind to a powder. Set aside in a small dish. Dry-roast the peppercorns in the same fashion, grind, and set aside in another small bowl. Place the salt in another dish and the coriander in another.

Place a non-stick fry pan or skillet over medium heat to preheat. Divide the dough into 8 equal pieces. With the palm of your hand, flatten each piece on a lightly floured surface, and set aside. (Do not stack.) Cover the dough with a cloth or plastic wrap to prevent drying out.

On a lightly floured surface, roll out one piece of dough into a 12-15 cm. circle. Sprinkle ¼ tspn cumin, a scant ¼ tspn ground pepper, ¼ tspn salt, and 1 tspn chopped coriander onto the dough. (At first you will want to use a measuring spoon. As you assemble subsequent breads, you will learn to judge the quantities by eye and feel, and the process will become smoother.)

Roll the dough up fairly tightly to give you a long cigar shape. Anchoring one end on your work surface, shape the bread into a flat coil, pressing the other end into the coil to make an even round. Flatten gently with the palm of your hand, then roll out to a circle about 12-15 cm. across and less than ½ cm. thick. Cook the bread for 1½ to 2 min. On the first side, or until lightly golden. Then turn and cook for 1 min. longer, until golden. Assemble and shape another bread while the first is cooking. Transfer the cooked bread to a cotton cloth and wrap to keep warm while you cook the remaining breads. Serve warm or at room temperature.

Puri

2 cups atta flour (or 2 cups whole wheat flour, sifted)
1½ cups sour light cream, or more as necessary
1 tspn freshly ground black pepper
1 tspn cumin seed, finely ground
1 tspn salt
½ tspn turmeric

In a medium-sized bowl, mix together the atta or wholewheat flour, pepper, cumin, turmeric, and salt. Add the sour light cream a little bit at a time, until a kneadable dough forms. The dough should be on the stiff side, but until easily kneadable; use less sour light cream as necessary. Turn the dough out onto a lightly floured surface and knead for 8 to 10 min. Return the bread to the bowl, cover, and let rest for 30 min. or as long as 2 hours.

Divide the dough into 16 balls of equal size. Flatten each ball between your lightly floured palms and set aside; do not stack. Cover with plastic wrap. Roll out each puri into a circle approximately 15 cm. in diameter. Set aside (do not stack them), and cover with plastic wrap.

These are usually deep fried but are just as yummy dry fried using a non stick pan. Cook over medium heat until golden brown on both sides.

Rava Dosa

2 cups semolina flour
1 cup sour light cream
½ tspn salt
2 cups warm water
1 tbsp finely chopped fresh ginger
1 red chilli pepper, seeded, de-veined, and finely chopped
2 tablespoons fresh coriander leaves, roughly chopped
1 tbsp fresh or dried curry leaves, if using dried, soak in water
for 10 min. before using

Rava dosas are thin crepe-like breads spiked with chillies, ginger, curry, and coriander leaves. In a medium-sized bowl, mix together the semolina flour, sour light cream, chilli, ginger, curry leaves, coriander leaves, and salt. Stir in the water a little bit at a time until you have a smooth batter. Cover the bowl and let the batter rest for approximately 1 hour.

Heat a non-stick pan over medium-high heat. When the frypan is hot, pour on ½ cup of the batter. As you pour, move in a circle out from the middle, distributing the batter in as large a circle as possible; then use the back of a wooden spoon or a rubber spatula to spread the batter to cover the gaps, again increasing the diameter of the dosa, to at least 23-25 cm. (Don't worry about making it too thin; the thinner the better.) Cook the dosa for 1½ min.; after cooking for 1 min. begin to loosen it from the pan with a spatula. Coax the dosa, don't force it, as it will come off easily when it is golden brown and ready. Flip to the other side and cook for 1½ to 2 min., or until lightly browned in spots. Remove to a plate. Continue cooking until all the dosas have been made. They can be stacked one on top of the other as they are cooked, or served immediately as they are made.

Unleavened Bread

Approx. 2 cups whole wheat flour
approx. 1 cup spring water

Preheat the oven to 180ºC. When the oven is hot, place 2 cups flour in a medium-sized bowl and stir in water until a kneadable dough forms; you may have to add a little more flour or water, depending on your flour. Turn the dough out onto a lightly floured surface and knead quickly and vigorously until smooth, about 3 to 4 min. Cut the dough into 12 equal pieces and flatten each into a round with lightly floured hands. Work with one piece of dough at a time, keeping the others covered with plastic wrap. On a lightly-floured surface, roll out one piece of dough as thin as possible. Prick it all over with a fork or a sharp-toothed comb, and then try to stretch it slightly to widen the holes you have made. Transfer to baking tray, placing it to one side to leave room for more breads and bake for 2½ to 3 min., until golden on the bottom and starting to crisp around the pricked holes.

Meanwhile, continue rolling out the dough, placing each bread in the oven, as it is ready. This will make it easier to get all the breads baked in time.

For traditional crisp, dried finish, leave the breads out on a rack to cool completely and to dry.

Unyeasted Date Cookies

1 cup warm water
1 tablespoon salt
4 cups date residue from Date Syrup (see recipe below)
6 to 7 cups hard whole wheat flour

In a medium-sized bowl, mix the warm water and salt. With a wooden spoon, stir in the date residue. Stir in the flour, a cup at a time, until the dough is too stiff to stir. Turn the dough out onto a floured surface and knead for 6 to 8 min., until relatively smooth and elastic, adding flour as necessary. Use a scraper to keep your work surface smooth and not too sticky. Cover with plastic wrap, and let rest for 30 min.

Place a rack in the centre of the oven, and preheat to 180ºC. Divide the dough into 2 equal pieces. Roll each piece out with a rolling pin on a well-floured surface until less than ½ cm. thick. Using a cookie cutter or a thin rimmed glass cut out shapes. Place the shapes on a dish.

Bake for 8 to 10 min. Place on racks to cool slightly, then wrap in a towel to keep warm; or alternatively, allow to cool completely and firm up.

Date Syrup

2½ kg pitted dates   8 cups boiling water

Wash the dates. Place the dates and boiling water in a large saucepan, stir well, and let stand to soak, covered, for 1 hour. Place the pan of dates over medium heat, and bring the water to a boil. Reduce the heat and simmer for 10 to 15 min. Remove from the heat and let cool.

Working with about 2 cups of the date mixture at a time, spoon the cooked dates into a large sieve or fine-mesh strainer placed over a large bowl and gently mash and press them against the mesh with a wooden spoon. Once most of the syrup has drained through from each batch, empty the colander, and set aside the date residue.

Store the date syrup in sterilised jars in the refrigerator, and use as a dip or as a sweetener; keeps well for up to 2 months. Makes approximately 5 cups of syrup.

Oasis Bread

4 cups unbleached all-purpose flour (extra for kneading)
2 tspns salt
2 cups warm water

Filling
1 tablespoon minced garlic
½ cup finely chopped eschallots (white and green parts)
1 small red capsicum, cored, seeded, and finely chopped
1½ cups drained canned tomatoes, coarsely chopped
½ tspn dried chilli pepper flakes, or more to taste
½ cup loosely packed flat-leafed parsley
½ tspn ground cumin and ground coriander
generous pinch of ground caraway
½ tspn salt

In a medium bowl, mix together the flour and salt. Make a well in the centre and slowly stir in the water until dough forms. Turn out onto a lightly floured surface and knead for 10 min. Clean out the bowl, place the dough back in the bowl, and cover with plastic wrap. Set aside. Heat a medium non-stick pan. Add the garlic and cook over medium-high heat stirring occasionally until it starts to brown. Add the eschallots and capsicum and cook, stirring for 2 min. or until slightly softened. Add the tomatoes and bring to a simmer. Reduce the heat to medium and simmer, stirring occasionally until the sauce thickens, about 15 min. Add the spices, chilli flakes and salt and simmer for 1 min. Stir in the parsley and transfer to a bowl. Let cool.

Working on a lightly floured surface, divide the dough into 8 pieces. Work with one piece at a time, keeping the others covered with plastic wrap.

Heat your pan over medium heat. Meanwhile, divide one piece of dough in half and flatten each with lightly-floured palms. Then roll out each piece to a circle approximately 15 cm. in diameter. Place 1 heaped tablespoon of the filling on the centre of one dough circle. Place the other circle on top and, with moistened fingers, pinch the edges together to seal well. Flatten gently, then stretch the bread out thinner by picking it up and stretching the edges, working all around the bread again to keep it round. Then hold the bread by two opposite *edges,* and pull your hands gently apart to stretch the bread further to a 20 cm diameter round.

Place in the hot frypan and cook for 1 min. then turn over and cook for 2 to 2½ min., until lightly speckled with brown on the bottom. Then turn over again and bake for 1 min. longer or until lightly browned. Remove from the skillet, fold in half, and wrap in a cotton cloth to keep warm and supple. Repeat with the remaining breads. Serve warm.

Cheese-filled Quick Bread

Cheese filling

30-35 g skim milk feta cheese, well crumbled (3-4 tbsps)
2 tbsps sour light cream

Dough
3 to 4 cups unbleached all-purpose flour
1½ tspns baking powder
½ tspn salt
2 cups sour light cream

Place an oven rack at the lowest position, and preheat the oven to 180ºC. To prepare the cheese filling: blend together all the ingredients in a bowl. Set aside. In a large bowl, mix together 1 cup flour, the baking powder, and salt. Add the sour light cream and stir well. Then continue stirring in flour until the dough has lost its stickiness and can be worked with your hands. Turn out onto a lightly floured surface and knead for 3 to 4 min., until soft and slightly elastic.

Divide the dough into 8 equal pieces. Keeping the remaining pieces covered with a cloth, work with one piece of dough at a time. Flatten the dough with the lightly-floured palm of your hand. Then, either stretching the dough or using a small rolling pin, flatten it out to a round about 15-20 cm. in diameter. Place 1 heaped tablespoon of the cheese filling in the centre of the dough. Pinch an edge of the dough between your thumb and forefinger and stretch it halfway over the filling to the centre of the dough round. Then pinch the edge an eighth of a turn along from the first position and bring it to the centre. Continue all the way around the circle, stretching the dough as you do so and pleating it over the filling until you have a dough-covered mound. Pinch the pleats closed and then with the lightly-floured palm of your hand, gently press down on the top of the mound to flatten it. Turn the bread over and gently press down again on the other side. This will push the filling out into the edges of the bread; it should be 5-10 mm. thick and 18-20 cm. in diameter.

Place the bread on a prepared baking tray and continue making breads until the first baking sheet is full. Bake the breads for 5 to 6 min., then remove from the oven, slide into a basket lined with a cloth, and cover to keep warm. Prepare the remainder of the breads while the first batch bakes, and then cook in the same fashion.

Paper Bread

1 cup coarse semolina (not flour) plus extra for dusting
1 cup unbleached white flour, plus extra for dusting
approx. ¾ cup warm water
¾ tspn salt

Place baking tray on the bottom rack of your oven and preheat oven to 180ºC. In a large bowl, mix together the semolina, flour, and salt. Stir in the water gradually, until the dough is smooth and no longer sticky. Form the dough into a ball and transfer to a well-floured work surface. Do not knead the dough.

Cut the dough in half, then cut each piece in half and then again to make 8 equal pieces. Roll each piece in the flour and/or semolina, then flatten with the floured palm of your hand. Roll out one piece at a time, keeping the remaining pieces covered with a cloth. Roll out one piece of dough as thin as possible on the lightly floured surface, rolling from the centre out and rotating the bread slightly between each stroke of your rolling pin. If the bottom starts to stick, flour the surface a little more and turn the bread over; you can also try flouring your rolling pin. You should aim for a bread less than 5 mm. thick, making a roughly circular bread 20-25 cm. across. Don't worry that the circle is not perfect.

After you finish rolling out the bread, transfer to a floured underside of a baking sheet, then slide gently onto the baking tray. Bake for 2 min., turn the bread over, and bake for 1 to 1½ min. longer. The bread should have golden spots and be crisp. Place it on a rack (or a window ledge) to dry out further.

Proceed to roll out and bake remaining breads in the same fashion, starting to roll out the next bread as soon as you place one in the oven. Eat warm or keep them for several weeks, stored in a dry place, and snack on them as you would on crackers.

Crackers

3-4 cups hard whole wheat flour, or more as necessary
2 tspns salt
½ cup warm water

Optional toppings
cayenne
coarse salt
cumin seed

Place the flour and salt in a food processor and process for 10 seconds to mix thoroughly. With the motor running, add the water in a steady stream, then process for 10 seconds longer. The dough should have formed into one large ball; if not, feel the dough. If it feels very sticky, add 3 to 4 tablespoons more flour and process briefly until a ball forms. If the dough feels dry and floury, start the processor again, add 2 to 3 tablespoons more water and process until a ball of dough forms.

Once you have a ball of dough, process for 1 min. Turn the dough out onto a lightly-floured surface and knead for 30 seconds or so. Cover with plastic wrap and let rest for 30 min.

Preheat the oven to 180ºC and place two racks near the centre of the oven. Divide the dough into 8 pieces. Work with one piece at a time, leaving the other pieces covered. On a lightly-floured surface, with lightly-floured hands, flatten a piece of dough with your palms. Then roll it out to a very thin rectangle or round, as even and thin as possible to ensure even cooking. Gently lift the dough from your rolling surface and place it on a large baking sheet or pizza pan. Sprinkle on one of the optional toppings or leave plain. Using a knife or a pizza cutter cut through the dough to make rectangular crackers. (Don't worry if they are not all exactly the same size.) Spray the dough lightly with water and place on the upper oven rack.

Begin rolling out the next piece of dough, keeping an eye on the crackers already baking. (Crackers brown from underneath.) Check on them 2½ to 3 min. after they go in. As soon as the thinnest patches of the dough have started to brown take them out. If necessary, continue baking, checking every 30 seconds, but it is better to take the crackers out a little early than too late.

You will soon get a feel for timing and degree of doneness. Variables that affect timing are the heat of your oven and how thin you managed to roll out your dough. When they come out of the oven, some of the crackers will be crisp, while others will need a little time in the air to crisp up. Transfer to a large bowl, breaking up any incompletely separated crackers. Roll out the remaining dough, season, and bake. When completely cool, crackers can be stored in a well-sealed plastic bag or cookie tins for up to a month.

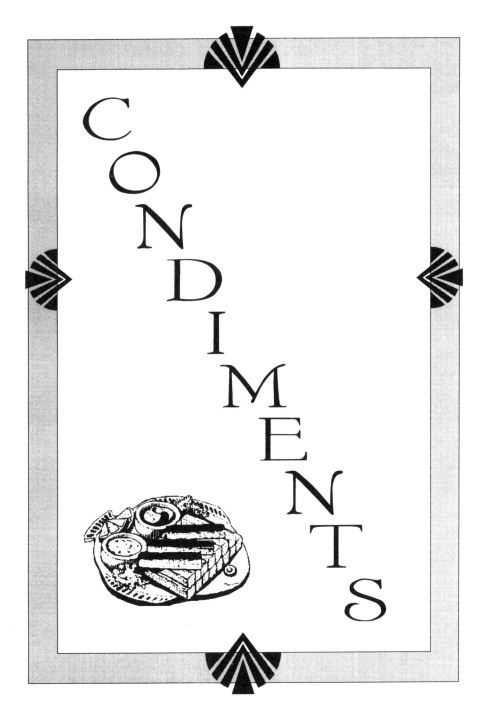

CONDIMENTS

Zeera Pani (Digestive: Cumin and Tamarind Water)

½ cup dried tamarind pulp
3 tspns grated ginger
pinch chilli powder
honey to taste
crushed ice, mint & lemon for serving

2 cups hot water
2 tspns ground cumin
½ tspn garam masala
salt to taste

A wonderful digestive to help at mealtimes. Soak tamarind in hot water and leave for 2 hours or overnight. Squeeze to dissolve pulp and separate seeds. Strain through sieve. Add remaining ingredients and stir well then strain through muslin cloth. Chill, dilute with ice water garnish and serve.

Chilli and Olive Spread

1 kg olives
1 tbsp crushed garlic
2 tbsps olive oil
350 g capers (drained if necessary)

1 tbsp grated ginger
2 tbsps chilli paste
1 cup vinegar

Place all the ingredients into a food processor and blend until smooth and well combined. Spoon the mixture into sterilised jars and seal. Use as a dressing for a fresh garden salad or with a tomato sauce to top some nice steamed vegetables

Chilli Salsa

5 tomatoes, chopped
1 jar chilli paste (see recipe)
1 bunch coriander, roughly chopped

2 cloves garlic, crushed
salt & pepper to taste

Cook onions for 2-3 min. until lightly cooked then add chilli and simmer for 2 min. Add the remaining ingredients and simmer for a further 10 min. Serve as a dip or sauce.

North African Chilli Paste

30 g dried hot red chillies (¾ cup), stems removed
½ tspn cumin seed, lightly dry roasted and ground
1½ tspns caraway seed, lightly dry-roasted
1 tspn coriander seed, lightly dry-roasted
4 to 6 cloves garlic, coarsely chopped
½ tspn salt, or to taste
olive oil

Soak the chillies in warm water for about 1 hour until they are soft. Drain and finely chop, discarding any hard bits. In a mortar, pound together the coriander, caraway, and cumin seed to a powder then add the garlic and salt and pound to a paste. Add the chillies and pound until broken down into a coarse paste. Then add enough olive oil to make a smooth paste.

Alternatively, grind the coriander, caraway, and cumin to a powder in a spice grinder. Then place the chillies, garlic, spices, and salt in a food processor or blender and process well, adding oil as necessary to blend into a smooth paste.

Mango Relish

4 kg mangoes, peeled and roughly chopped
6 medium onions finely chopped
small knob of ginger, finely grated
juice of 3 limes & 1 lemon
pinch of cloves

1½ tbsps ground cinnamon

5 tspns ground allspice

1-1½ cups vinegar

4 cups honey

Mix all ingredients in a large pot and bring to the boil then simmer for 60-90 min. Add extra spices or honey as required by taste (the honey and vinegar should balance out, i.e., the vinegar should not make you gag but it should not be too sweet). Pour into sterilised jars, allow to cool and store in dark and cool cupboard. Refrigerate when opened.

Spicy Tomato Chutney

2 large tomatoes (about 500 g), coarsely chopped
1½ tbsps minced garlic, (approximately 4 medium cloves)
1 cup loosely packed fresh coriander, coarsely chopped
½ tspn fenugreek seed, dry-roasted and ground
½ tspn cumin seed, dry-roasted and ground
1 tbsp finely chopped fresh ginger
1 medium onion, finely chopped
1 tbsp vegetable oil
3 fresh green chillies chopped
½ tspn salt

Heat a non-stick pan over a medium high heat. Add the garlic, onion, ginger, and chillies and fry for 1 min. Add the fenugreek and cumin and cook 1 min. more, stirring. Add the tomatoes and salt, and bring to a boil. Lower the heat, partially cover, and cook for another 15 min. or until thickened almost to a paste.

Turn out into a bowl and stir in the coriander leaves. Serve as a condiment and dipping sauce for bread. Stored in the refrigerator, well sealed in a glass container. It will keep for a week.

Green Chilli Chutney

1 cup loosely packed fresh coriander leaves, finely chopped
½ cup loosely packed fresh mint leaves, finely chopped
4 green chillies, finely chopped
pinch of asafoetida
½ tspn cumin seed, dry-roasted
¼ tspn salt
2 tbsps fresh lemon juice

Add all the ingredients except the lemon juice and pound until you
have a mash. Add the lemon juice and continue to pound until a
slightly dry paste forms. Alternatively, combine all the ingredients
in a food processor and process briefly to blend; you want a slightly
rough paste, not a uniform texture. This is best eaten immediately,
or within 2 to 3 hours, while the fresh herbs until have good flavour.

Peach Chutney

2 kg ripe peaches, peeled and quartered
½ cup vinegar
¾ cup honey   2 tspns cinnamon

Place all ingredients into a large pan and simmer for 1 hour, or
until mixture is thick, stirring often.
        Spoon into sterilised jars and seal while hot.

Tomato Relish

1 kg tomatoes, skinned and roughly chopped
5-6 red capsicums or yellow peppers roughly chopped
½ tspn mustard powder   ½ cup vinegar

4 onions, roughly chopped
½ cup honey½ tspn cayenne

1 tbsp curry powder
¼ cup salt

Put tomatoes, onion and peppers in pot and mix well. Sprinkle the salt on top and leave to stand overnight. Next morning drain off the juice (keep in fridge and have as a refreshing tomato juice), add the remaining ingredients, bring to the boil and then simmer for 1 hour until most of the liquid has evaporated. Spoon into sterilised jars and store in cool, dark cupboard until required. Refrigerate after opening.

Green Tomato Chutney

6 large green tomatoes
6 medium chokos (sliced)
300-400 ml apple cider vinegar
1 tspn ground cloves
handful sea salt

6 large onions
500g honey
1 tspn cayenne powder
2 tspns cinnamon

Slice tomato, sprinkle with the sea salt and leave to stand overnight. Next day boil, using the juice formed. When at boiling point add the remaining ingredients and cook until tender. Place in sterile jars, allow to cool and store.

Chilli Paste

100 g chillies
1 red capsicum
1 tbsp vinegar
2 tbsps coriander
1 tspn fenugreek
2 tbsps honey

4 cloves garlic
2 tbsps tamari
1 onion
1 tspn paprika
¼ cup water

Roughly chop all ingredients and place them all (except the honey) in the blender. Blend until you have a fairly smooth consistency. Place all the ingredients in a pot, add the honey and bring to the boil then simmer for 10 min. Place chilli paste in jar, allow to cool then refrigerate.

Pickled Onions

2 kg small pickling onions
2 litres apple cider vinegar
2 cups rock salt
bay leaves, red chillies, coloured peppercorns

2½ litres water
1 cup honey

Peel and trim the onions, place into a bowl with water and salt and soak for 24 hours. Make sure you use a non-metallic container or a plastic bucket. Drain the onions, then pack them into jars with the bay leaves, red chillies and peppercorns.

Bring the vinegar and honey to boil and pour over the onions. Cover and store for 3-4 weeks before using (If you can wait).

Beetroot Relish

1 kg beetroots peeled and finely grated or shredded
2 onions, finely chopped
1 cup vinegar
½ cup honey
1 tspn mixed spice

Sauté onion in pan over a low heat for 5 min. then add beetroot and cook for a further 10 min. Add remaining ingredients and mix well. Simmer for 45 min. or until mixture is thick and beetroot is tender. Spoon into sterilised jars and seal while hot.

SAUCES

Soya Cheese Sauce

100 g soya cheese
2 tbsps tamari
shake of paprika & cumin
½ cup water or vegetable stock

½ tspn crushed garlic
juice of ¼ lemon
salt & pepper to taste

Slowly melt cheese in a non-stick pot over a low heat. Add remaining ingredients except the water and mix together. Add water a bit at a time until you have the required consistency. Use with, lightly steamed, fresh vegetables.

Spicy Tomato Sauce

2 kg tomatoes skinned & pureed
2 onions, finely chopped
2 cloves garlic, crushed
½ cup honey
1 tspn cloves
½ tspn chilli paste
¼ tspn black pepper

1 tbsp salt
½ cup vinegar
½ tspn ground allspice
1 tspn curry powder
1 tspn paprika
pinch cayenne

Mix all ingredients in a large pot and bring to the boil then simmer until the consistency is of a tomato sauce. Pour into sterilised jars, allow to cool and store in dark and cool cupboard. Refrigerate when opened.

Miso Sauce

1 tbsp miso dissolved in some warm water
2 tbsps tomato paste

2 cups water
1 eschallot finely chopped
1 onion, finely chopped
1 stick celery, finely chopped
3 cloves garlic, crushed
½ cup finely chopped mint, coriander, basil

Sauté onion, garlic and eschallots until they start to brown and onion becomes translucent. Add the rest of the ingredients and bring to boil then simmer for 4-5 min.

Cream Curry Sauce

3 tbsps sour light cream
2-3 tbsps curry powder

1 tbsp honey
2-3 tbsps tamari

Mix ingredients well and heat until bubbling. Presto ready to go over those beautiful vegetables.

Cashew and Mushroom Sauce

¼ cup raw cashews, crushed
1 cup water
½ cup mushrooms chopped
1 tbsp tamari
¼ tspn cinnamon

Blend all the ingredients together and cook, over low heat, until mixture is smooth and creamy. Serve hot or cold over any vegetable dishes.

Hot Mexican Sauce

4 tomatoes, chopped   ¾ cup olives, pitted
¼ cup hot peppers, minced   1 tbsp tamari
1 tspn fenugreek powder   ¼ cup basil, chopped

Combine all ingredients together and allow to stand in fridge for an hour so that the flavours blend. Serve at room temperature over vegetables or as garnish for a salad. May also be used as dip.

Leek Sauce

2-4 leeks   2-4 tbsps oil
2-4 tbsps water   1 tspn basil
1 tspn thyme   1 tspn parsley

Cut leeks into slices and steam until soft then place in blender with the rest of the ingredients and puree. Pour over cooked vegetables. Do not heat this dish as it contains oil.

Mushroom Sauce

250 g mushrooms   1 medium onion
½ capsicum   2 eschallots
2 cloves garlic   1 tspn grated ginger
2 medium tomatoes   1 zucchini
1 carrot   2 tbsps tamari
1 cup water   salt & pepper
1 cup freshly chopped coriander, mint, parsley

Dry fry the onion, garlic and ginger then add the other ingredients, which have been previously chopped into small pieces, and bring to boil. Simmer for 5-10 min. then puree in blender and pour over steamed vegetables of your choice.

Nutty Garlic and Ginger Sauce

1 tbsp ginger & garlic finely chopped	6 mushrooms
50 g almond meal	1 eschallot
1 onion finely chopped	1 tspn miso
4 tomatoes skinned	1 tbsp cinnamon
2 tbsps tamari	2 tbsps vinegar
1 tspn hot paprika	¼ cup lemon

To skin tomatoes place them in boiling water until the skin starts to come off, then peel. Sauté onions, garlic, ginger and eschallots in the tamari and vinegar. Add hot paprika, cinnamon, mushrooms and half the almond meal while continuing to stir well. Add tomatoes, chopped, and lemon then allow mixture to simmer for 5 min. before adding the rest of the almond meal. At any stage you may thin with boiling water. This sauce is ideal for pouring over Steamed Minted Cauliflower.

Onion Sauce

2 medium onion	2 tbsps tomato paste
1 tspn cumin	1 tspn fenugreek powder
2 cups water	

Sauté ingredients until onion becomes translucent then add the water and simmer for 10 min. Pour over steamed vegetables, fish etc.

DRESSING AND MARINADES

Berry Vinegars

300 g berries
750 ml vinegar

Place berries into a jar large enough to hold the vinegar as well and seal the jar. Store for about three months then strain vinegar from the berries and pour it into sterilised bottles to use as required.

Note: All types of berries work well in this recipe.

Tomato and Garlic Marinade

¼ cup tomato paste
1 clove garlic, crushed
juice & grated rind of 1 medium lemon
1 tspn honey

Combine all ingredients together and use as a marinade, or as a brushing sauce for chicken or seafood dishes.

Coriander Vinaigrette

½ small onion, thinly sliced
1 tspn wholegrain mustard
½ cup oil (use your preferred oil)

1 tspn coriander seeds
2 tbsps vinegar

In a frying pan over heat, cook the coriander seeds, stirring continuously for 2 min. When they become fragrant remove from the heat. Grind them into a powder using mortar and pestle or any other grinding implement. In a bowl whisk the vinegar, mustard and coriander.

Dribble this into the oil via a thin stream until all the ingredients are well mixed. Add onions and salt and pepper to taste. Stir well before pouring.

Herb Dressing

¼ cup finely chopped fresh herbs
— basil, thyme, garlic chives, mint
2 cloves garlic, finely chopped

$\frac{1}{3}$ cup vinegar	1 cup oil
juice of ½ lemon	¼ cup tamari
1 tspn, onion powder	1 tspn, paprika
½ tspn, cumin	2 drops tabasco sauce
2 tbsps honey	salt & pepper to taste

The oil used can be any of your favourites, i.e., corn, olive, grapeseed, etc. Place all ingredients into a tall container and blend with mixer. Adjust ingredients to taste and serve over wonderful vegetables and salad. Makes about 700-750 mls.

Vindaloo Marinade

1 tspn ground chilli powder	¼ cup vinegar
1 tspn ground cardamom	1 tspn ground cinnamon
2 tspns ground turmeric	2 tbsps honey
2 tspns dry mustard	2 tspns ground cumin

Combine all ingredients together and use as a marinade, or as a brushing sauce for chicken or seafood dishes.

Avocado Dressing

1-2 medium avocados
4 tbsps tamari
fresh ground black pepper
2 cloves garlic, crushed

2 tbsps tomato paste
½ cup lemon juice
4 tbsps vinegar

Mix all ingredients together (by hand or in blender) and mix into fresh garden salad.

Miso and Ginger Dressing

2 tbsps miso
¼ cup vinegar

2 tbsps ginger, grated
½ cup water

Blend the miso, ginger and vinegar together and slowly add the water until the dressing is thick and creamy. Adjust any flavours to taste and refrigerate. Ideal for steamed vegetables or grated carrot and spinach salad.

Mustard Dressing

1 tbsp each of yellow & brown mustard
1 onion finely chopped
2 cloves garlic
2 tspns fenugreek powder
2 tspns cumin

3 tbsps vinegar
¼ cup water
3 tbsps oil, optional

Place all ingredients in blender and mix until smooth. Season to taste and store in fridge until required.

If using oil do not use where dish contains other fatty acid/starch/protein.

Spicy Dressing/Marinade

½ cup lemon juice   ½ cup vinegar
2 cloves garlic   salt & pepper to taste
1 tspn cardamom powder   1 tspn hot paprika
sprinkle of oregano & thyme   2 tbsps tamari

Mix all ingredients together thoroughly. May be used for a salad dressing or a marinade for fish, chicken, etc.

Tahini Dressing

½ cup tahini   2 cloves garlic
½ cup lemon juice   1 tspn tamari
1 tbsp parsley chopped   1 tspn honey
pinch cayenne & paprika   1 tspn ground cumin

Blend all ingredients together and serve with salad or steamed vegetables. No other protein, starch or fatty acid.

Refrigerate if necessary and use as required.

Tangy Dressing

2 tomatoes, chopped   2 cloves garlic, crushed
2 tbsps tamari   1 tbsp oregano
1 tbsp basil, 1 cup oil

Using a blender or food processor mix together all the ingredients until they are well combined.

Refrigerate and use as required.

BASIC DRESSINGS

150 mls low fat sour light cream   salt & pepper to taste
2 cloves garlic, crushed   2 tbsps lemon juice

Place sour light cream in a bowl and beat until smooth. Add remainder of ingredients and mix well.

Variations

Honey
stir in 2 tspns of honey

Honey and Mint
as above with 1 tbsp mint finely chopped

Honey and Lime
as for the basic dressing but use lime instead of lemon

Horseradish
add 2 tbsps grated horseradish

Mustard
add 1-2 tbsps coarse grained mustard (see page:23) and 1 tbsp fresh dill

CURRIES

Garam Masala

½ cup black peppercorns   ½ cup coriander seed
½ cup cumin seed   2 tbsps cloves

one 5 cm. cinnamon stick, broken into pieces
1 tbsps green cardamom seeds

Heat a non-stick pan over medium-high heat. Add all the ingredients and dry roast, stirring constantly with a wooden spoon, for 3 to 4 min., or until the spices start to give off an aroma. Keep stirring for 2 min. more then remove from the heat and transfer to a bowl. Let cool.

In a spice grinder, grind the roasted spices to a powder. Let cool completely. Store in a glass jar. Well-sealed in a glass jar, garam masala keeps indefinitely, though the vigour of the flavours will decline after several months.

Mango Curry

3 ripe medium mangoes, peeled & cut into ¾-inch cubes
2 green or red chillies, finely chopped
1 tbsp tamarind paste or pulp
1 small onion, coarsely chopped
½ tspn black mustard seed
1 clove garlic, coarsely chopped
½ tspn cumin seed, dry-roasted
½ cup hot water

½ tspn turmeric
1 cup warm water
1 tbsp palm sugar
½ tspn salt

In a small bowl, dissolve the tamarind paste or pulp in the hot water and stir well. If using pulp, press the seeds to detach the flesh, and strain through a sieve into another bowl, pressing the pulp against the mesh with a spoon to extract the maximum from the tamarind; discard the pulp. Set the syrupy tamarind water aside.

In a large mortar, pound the cumin seed to a powder. Add the garlic, onion, and salt and pound to a paste. Alternatively,

185

use a spice grinder to grind the cumin. Then combine the cumin, garlic, onion, and salt in a food processor and process to a paste.

Dissolve the palm sugar in the warm water in a small bowl, and stir in the reserved tamarind water. In a non-stick pan add the mustard seeds and cook over medium heat until they pop (cover with the lid as they begin to pop).

Add the cumin paste and cook, stirring constantly until it begins to brown slightly. Add the tamarind mixture, together with the mangoes, chillies, and turmeric.

Raise the heat and bring to a boil, then lower the heat to medium and simmer for 10 to 15 min., until thickened.

Green Curry Paste

4 large fresh green chillies (use red chillies for red paste)
2 tbsps chopped fresh coriander plant, including root
1 small brown onion finely chopped
1 tbsp garlic finely chopped
1 tspn black peppercorns
2 tspns chopped lemon rind
2 tspns ground coriander
1 tspn cumin powder
2 tspns dried shrimp powder
1 tspn ground turmeric

1 tbsp oil or tamari
1 tspn salt
1 tspn serai powder
1 tspn laos powder
2 tspns paprika

The serai, laos and shrimp powder can be found in most Asian stores. Blend all ingredients together and add to your favourite vegetable and chicken or fish dishes.

Note: If you use the oil in this dish then do not mix with other proteins, starches or fatty acids

Eastern Curry Paste

5 cardamom pods or ½ tspn ground cardamom
1 stick cinnamon or 1 tspn ground cinnamon
7-10 dried chillies or 2 tspns chilli powder
5 whole cloves or ¼ tspn ground cloves
1 tspn shredded lemon grass

2 tbsps coriander powder | 1 tspn cumin powder
2 medium onions finely chopped | 2 tspns laos powder
5 cloves garlic, thinly sliced | ½ tspn ground mace
½ tspn dried shrimp paste | 1 tspn fennel powder

Roast chillies in dry pan and pound in mortar and pestle. Roast coriander seeds in dry pan and pound in mortar and pestle. Roast cumin seeds in dry pan and pound in mortar and pestle. Add laos and lemon grass to ground spices. Roast cloves, cinnamon stick, cardamom pods and mace then grind in mortar and pestle. Combine all spices and set aside. Stir-fry onion, garlic and shrimp paste for 1-2 min. (If using ground spices only dry roast the coriander and fennel.) Combine all ingredients to form a paste.

Nam Prik

2 tbsps dried shrimps | 1½ tbsps tamari
1 tspn dried shrimp paste | 2 tspns ground chilli
4 cloves garlic, crushed | 3 tbsps water
2 tspns palm sugar | 2 tbsps lemon juice

Wash shrimps and soak in hot water for 20 min. then rinse. Wrap dried shrimp paste in aluminium foil and put under a hot grill for 3 min. either side. Put all ingredients in blender and blend to paste.

DIPS

Tzatziki (Greek Garlic Dip)

500 g sour light cream
juice of ½ a lemon
1 medium Lebanese cucumber
¼ cup finely chopped mint
4-5 cloves garlic, crushed

2 tspns hot paprika
2 tbsps vinegar
2 tspns cumin
juice of ½ a lemon
salt & pepper to taste

Finely grate cucumber and strain of the excess liquid. Mix in with all the other ingredients and allow to stand in fridge for 1-2 hours. Serve with crunchy vegetable sticks on a hot summer's day.

Avocado Dip

1-2 medium avocados
4 tbsps tamari
4 tbsps vinegar
fresh ground black pepper

2 tbsps tomato paste
½ cup lemon juice
2 cloves garlic, crushed

Blend all ingredients together until the taste is as desired. Serve with vegetable sticks and a crisp garden salad with a lemon dressing.

Eggplant and Capsicum Dip

2 eggplants
1 tbsp capers, chopped
1 stick celery, finely chopped
2 tbsps parsley, chopped
1 tspn salt

2 capsicums red
2 tbsps oil
2 tspns vinegar
2 cloves garlic, crushed
1 tspn cayenne

Preheat the oven to 200ºC. Pierce the eggplant skins with a fork and place with the capsicums directly on the oven rack with a tray underneath to catch any juices. While they are cooking combine together all the ingredients in a large bowl.

When the peppers blister (about 20 min.) remove them from the oven and cool for 5 min. Peel, seed and chop before adding them to the bowl. The eggplants take about 45 min. before done. When ready scoop out the pulp, chop finely and add to bowl also with any juices you have collected. Allow to sit overnight before serving.

Greek Garlic Dip

6-8 cloves garlic, crushed
1 tspn salt
2-3 tbsps lemon juice
¼-½ cup water

4 potatoes, cubed
½ cup parsley, chopped
1 tbsp sour light cream

Steam potatoes until soft and mash together with the sour light cream. Stir in the rest of the ingredients and add lemon to taste. Slowly mix in enough water to make the dip a creamy texture. May be used as dip or sauce over steamed vegetables.

Smoked Eggplant Dip

2 medium eggplants, very ripe
½ lemon, juice
1 tbsp sour light cream

3 cloves garlic, crushed
salt & pepper to taste

Wrap eggplant in foil and cook in enclosed fire for ½ hr (fuel stove). Slice eggplant in half and scoop out flesh ensuring you scrape the skin to get the smoked flavour. Put ingredients in blender and blend until smooth. Garnish with paprika and serve with chopped vegetables or salad.

Tomato and Chilli Dip

4 tbsps tomato paste
1 tspn cumin
2 cloves garlic, crushed
2 tbsps water

1 tspn chilli paste
2 tbsps tamari
1 tbsps garam masala

Mix ingredients together in bowl and serve with fresh, crisp vegies or with fish pieces lightly dry fried.

Tahini and Mint Dip

½ cup tahini
2 tbsps sour light cream
fresh mint to taste

2 lemons, juice
3 cloves garlic

Blend together all ingredients and allow to sit for 1 hour. Spoon some over salad or steamed vegetables. Chill the rest until required.

MUSTARDS

For all the following dressings place all ingredients in a jar and shake well until combined or mix with a spoon in a bowl. If these dressings are to be used for vegetables or salad you may add oil if desired but remember not to mix with any other protein starch or fatty acid.

If you do not like the texture of the mustard seeds then use mustard powder instead. Piquancy increases if left for a few days.

The longer the better. Also the more you cook any mustard the milder it becomes.

Coarse Grained Mustard

1 cup yellow or black mustard seeds or both (about 100g)
2 tspns finely chopped herbs of your choice
½ cup vinegar or herb vinegar
1 tspn black peppercorns
½ cup water
2 tbsps honey
1 tbsp salt

Roughly grind mustard seeds and peppercorns and combine with other ingredients. Mix well, use a hand blender if necessary.

Hot Chilli Mustard

1 tbsp yellow mustard seeds, finely ground
1 tbsp black/brown mustard seeds, finely ground
3 small dried red chilli peppers, very finely chopped
1 tbsp mustard powder
1 clove garlic, crushed
1 tbsp fresh lime juice
salt & pepper to taste

Pineapple And Chilli Mustard

May be made without the chilli if you so desire. Also cherries make a wonderfully flavoured mustard.

3 tbsps mustard powder   1 tspn chilli powder

125 g chopped pineapple
1 tspn salt
1 tspn thyme

1 tbsp sherry
1 tspn dried oregano

Citrus Mustard

2 tbsps yellow & brown mustard seeds, coarsely ground
1 lemon & 1 lime zest & juice only
2 tbsps honey

MUSTARD VARIATIONS
(Combine ingredients in small bowl)

Garlic Mustard

1 head garlic, roasted (wrapped in foil and roast at 200°C for
30 min., then carefully squeeze out the softened garlic.)
5 tbsps prepared mustard (see above)
freshly ground black pepper
1 eschallot finely chopped

Olive Mustard

5 tbsps prepared mustard
15 pitted black olives, finely chopped

1 tbsp olive paste
1 tbsp olive oil

Ginger and Coriander

5 tbsps prepared mustard
1 clove garlic,
1 cm. piece fresh ginger root, finely chopped
½ cup fresh coriander leaves, finely chopped

Dill Mustard

5 tbsps prepared mustard
1 tbsp sour light cream
2 tbsps freshly chopped dill
freshly ground black pepper

Sun-dried Tomato Mustard

1 tbsp chopped fresh tarragon
5 tbsps prepared mustard
45 g sun-dried tomatoes puréed in 2 tbsps water

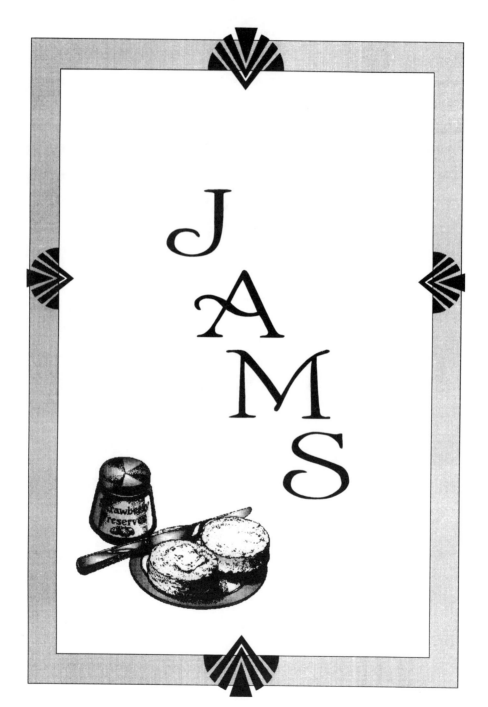

JAMS

Carrot Jam

1 kg carrots
600 g honey
4 lemons
1 cup water

Wash and finely grate carrots. Halve lemons, remove seeds and chop in food processor or alternatively slice very thinly. Combine carrots, lemons and water and allow to stand overnight.

Bring to the boil and continue boiling until soft. Add honey and boil rapidly until mixture thickens. Pour into sterilised jars and allow to cool before sealing.

Apricot Marmalade

3 kg of halved and pipped apricots
750 g fresh pineapple, finely chopped and cored
1.5 kg honey juice of 1 lemon
½ cup water

Put the apricots, pineapple and water in a large pot and boil until they just start to release their juices. Be careful as they stick easily so stir regularly with a wooden spoon. Turn off heat, cover and leave for 3-4 hours.

Bring to the boil again over a slow flame, stirring often until it starts to thicken then add the honey and boil until it thickens to a good consistency, i.e., fairly thick. Add the lemon juice, stir in while boiling for a few min. then take off the flame. Place jam in jars, seal and allow to cool before storing.

Mixed Berry Jam

1.5 kg mixed berries
¼ cup lemon juice
shredded rind of a lemon

¼ cup water
750 g honey

Place berries, water, juice and rind into a large pan and simmer for 15 min. Add the honey and stir in. Boil for about 40 min., stirring occasionally until the mixture reaches setting point (see Appendix).

Raspberry Jam

3 cups raspberries
1.75 cups honey
1 green apple, cored and roughly chopped

Prepare the raspberries by taking off the stems and place them in a saucepan with the apples and honey. Slowly bring to the boil then simmer for about 1-1½ hours until the jam takes on a solid consistency. Place in sterilised jars and seal while hot. Allow to cool then store in cupboard. Refrigerate after opening.

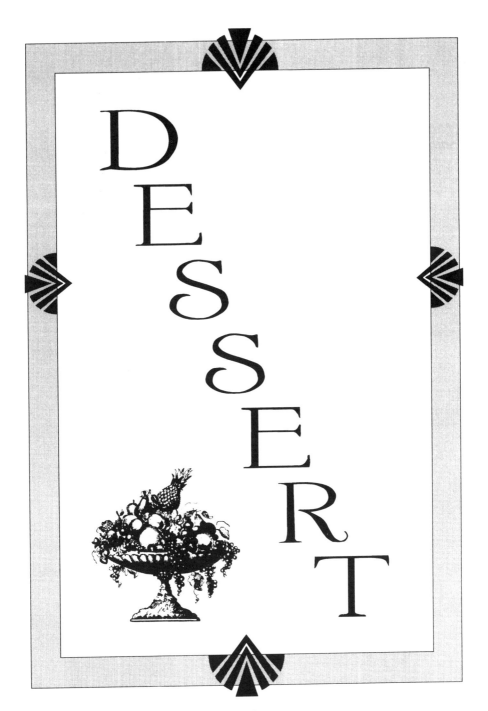

DESSERT

Oatmeal Rookies

4 cups instant oats
½ cup apple juice concentrate
2 tspns ginger powder
3 tspns cinnamon powder
¼ tspn sea salt
2 tspns aniseed powder

2 cups oat meal
1 tspn vanilla essence
1 cup honey (melted)
2 tspns baking powder
1 tspn ground cloves
½ tspn allspice powder

2 tbsps apple paste (or 100 g dried apple pieces soaked in 200 ml hot water)

Optional
3 drops Angostura bitters
1 tspn Vit. C powder

Mix all ingredients together to form a thick paste. Spoon mixture onto a non-stick tray, or into paper patty cups (make to whatever size you desire) and place into a pre heated oven, 100°C, for about 15-20 min.

Almond Cookies

2 cups almond meal
½ cup honey (heated until runny)
1 tspn cinnamon
½ tspn allspice
500 g sour light cream, extra light

2 tspns baking powder
1 tbsp vanilla essence
½ tspn ginger powder
1 tspn vinegar

Pre heat oven to 100°C. Combine all the ingredients together and mix. Place in cookie tray or into paper patty cups and cook for 10-15 min. until golden brown. Allow to cool then remove from tray.

Apple Turnovers

The dough is a simple flatbread dough-flour, salt, and water –
no oil, no flaky pastry, just a straightforward, taste of wheat.

1 kg apples (preferably Delicious)
2 cups whole wheat flour
1 cup unbleached white flour
1 tbsp ground cinnamon
½ cup apple juice or water

1½ cups water
½ cup brown honey
1 tspn salt
juice of 1 lime

In a medium-sized bowl, mix together the flours and salt. Make a
well in the centre and pour in the water. Stir vigorously in one
direction until all the flour is absorbed. This helps keep together
the gluten strands. When the dough becomes too stiff to stir,
turn it onto a lightly floured breadboard. Knead for 5 min., adding
more flour if the dough is sticky. Cover with plastic wrap and let
rest for 30 min.

Cut the apples into small chunks (peel or don't peel as you
like). In a medium bowl, mix the apples with the honey, cinnamon,
lime juice and apple juice or water. Mix well. Position a rack in the
centre of the oven, and preheat the oven to 180ºC. Divide the
dough into 12 equal pieces. Between floured palms, pat each piece
into a flat disc. With a rolling pin, roll out each disc until
approximately 20 cm.in diameter. If the dough is too soft and
sticky, use flour to help in rolling. Put half a cup of the apple mixture
just slightly off-centre on each round. Fold the dough in half to
enclose the apple mixture, creating a turnover. Pinch together
the edges and flute in a decorative way. (If the edges are not
tightly sealed, some of the apple filling will ooze out during baking.)

Arrange the turnovers on the baking sheets and bake for
20 to 25 min. Cool on a rack before serving.

Berry Cakes

3 cups unbleached all-purpose flour
1 tspn salt   1 tbsp baking powder
1 cup fresh blueberries   1½ cups water

If blueberries are unavailable, substitute other berries, fresh or frozen, and balance their tartness by adding honey.

In a bowl, mix the flour, salt, and baking powder until thoroughly blended. Add the berries (or berries and honey) and stir to mix in. Make a well in the middle of the dry ingredients, pour in the water and stir quickly to mix. The dough should be fairly stiff but evenly moistened.

Transfer the batter to the non-stick pan. With wet fingers, lightly pat out the batter to fill the skillet. Place in the centre of the oven and bake for 20 to 25 min. or until it is firm to the touch in the centre. Carefully remove it from the skillet and transfer to a rack to cool. Serve warm or at room temperature.

Buckwheat Cake/Drop-Cakes

2 cups buckwheat flour   ½ cup honey
¼ cup hot water   1 tbsp vinegar
2 tspns baking powder   ½ tspn nutmeg powder
2 tspns vanilla essence   ½ tspn lemon juice
1 tspn cinnamon powder   1 tspn ginger powder
½ tspn all spice powder

Put the flour into a large dish, sift in the baking powder then add all the spices and mix well. Combine all the liquid ingredients together and add to the flour mixture and start to mix it all together. When the ingredients have been thoroughly mixed together place the mixture in a cake tin which has been lined with foil. Cook at about 160º-180ºC until the mixture has cooked through (usually about 20 min.).

As an alternative, the mixture can be spooned into paper cup cake holders and become drop cakes. Cook for less time.

Ginger Biscuits

1 cup buckwheat flour	1 tspn baking powder
¼ cup warm water	¼ cup honey
fresh ginger and nutmeg to taste	1 tbsp apple cider vinegar

Mix all ingredients together and bake in a moderate oven (preheated to 180ºC) for about 10-15 min. in a cookie tray.

Carrot Cake

1 cup wholemeal flour	1 tspn baking powder
1 tspn cinnamon	1½ cup grated carrot
½ cup honey	¼ cup water

Preheat oven to 180ºC. Combine honey and water until thoroughly mixed. Stir in dry ingredients, carrots. Bake in rectangular tin for 20-30 min.

Moist Apple Cake/Banana Cake

2 tspns cinnamon	2 cups flour
1 apple, cored or banana pureed	1 cup honey
2 tspns vanilla essence (see recipe)	½ tspn rock salt
1 tspn baking powder (see recipe)	
3 cups finely cored and chopped apples or banana	

Preheat oven to 180°C. In a medium bowl mix flour, baking powder, cinnamon and salt. When these are well mixed add the apples, mix and place in a dish with a layer of greaseproof paper or foil on the bottom. Bake for 45-55 min. or until done. This is one of these recipes you will need to play around with until you get it to your liking. Add other spices, have fun, experiment.

Fruit Compote with Scented Waters

250 g unsulfured dried apricots (about 2 cups)
100 g pitted prunes (about ¾ cup)
2 tbsps honey, or more to taste   1 tbsp fresh lemon juice
100 g raisins (about ¾ cup)   1 tspn rose water
1 tspn orange blossom water   1½ cups water

You will need a large non-reactive bowl and a small bowl. Rinse the fruit quickly, and place in a non-reactive bowl. In a small bowl, mix the honey, water, and rose and orange waters. Pour over the fruit. Let stand for at least 24 or up to 48 hours, covered, in a cool place or in the refrigerator. Just before serving, stir in the lemon juice. Taste, and sprinkle on an extra tbsp or more of honey if you wish. Serve at room temperature, in a glass serving bowl.

Crystallised Rinds

4 cups prepared rinds   500-750 g honey
½-1 cup water   1 lemon sliced

To prepare the rinds remove the pith and skin of the citrus fruits making sure that no flesh is included. If using watermelon, leave 5 mm of the white flesh attached.

Cut the prepared rind into thick strips and place into a pan, cover with water and simmer for 20 min., drain well. Place honey and water into pan and mix thoroughly. Add rind and lemon, simmer for 1 hour over a very low heat until the syrup is really thick. Remove the rind from the syrup and allow to cool on a rack before placing in an airtight container.

Cherry Ice-cream

250 g fresh cherries, pitted
750 g extra light sour light cream

1 tspn vanilla essence
½ cup honey

Place all ingredients except a few cherries in a non-stick saucepan over a low flame, stir often. Once bubbling allow to simmer for 10 min., stirring often. Pour into loaf tin, microwave or non stick. Put into freezer until chilled then using a hand blender stir until fluffy then freeze.

Fresh Fruit Jelly

2¼ cups of juice, freshly squeezed and strained
3 tspns gelatine or agar powder
chopped fruit pieces
¼ cup honey
¼ cup cold water

Combine juice and honey in pan and stir over low heat until honey has dissolved. Sprinkle gelatine over cold water and allow to stand for 1-2 min. until the granules have expanded then mix in. If they do not dissolve stir mixture over hot water. Add to the hot liquid in the pan, stir and allow to cool away from the heat.

Place fruit pieces into glass or bowl, the pieces should float and refrigerate until the mixture is set.

Berry Mousse

2 cups berry puree (any berry that is available)
3 tspn gelatine or agar powder
¼ cup cold water　　　　　　2 tbsps honey
2 tspns grated citrus rind　　1 cup sour light cream

Sprinkle gelatine or agar over the cold water, stir over hot water until dissolved. Add berry puree and rind and chill until almost set. Mix honey with the sour light cream and lightly whip then fold through the berry mixture and spoon into individual glasses. Chill until set.

Soy Milk Sorbet

3 cups soy milk (unsweetened soy milk with no added oils, rice bran, etc.)
½ cup honey heated until liquid　　1 tspn cinnamon
3 tbsps vanilla essence

Blend together all the ingredients for 30 sec. then pour in container and freeze. After an hour or two as it just starts to harden take out and blend once more then refreeze.

For the kids, freeze in plastic cups with icy-pole sticks so they can have a healthy snack.

Sago Pudding

4 tbsps sago (soaked in 1 cup cold water)
juice of 2-3 medium sized lemons
rind of 1 lemon grated
4 tbsps maple syrup (the pure one not the pretend one)

Add the sago, 2 cups of water and the remaining ingredients to a pot, stir continuously and bring to the boil. It should be the consistency of clear jelly. Pour into wet mould and allow to cool and set. Garnish with a dash of cinnamon and serve.

Pineapple Buckwheat Pancakes

1½ cups buckwheat flour
½ tspn baking powder
½ tspn cinnamon powder
maple syrup, 100% pure
pineapple (unsweetened) pieces, drain the juice and use to mix batter to smooth consistency

½ cup skim milk powder
2 tbsps honey

Mix all ingredients, except maple syrup and pineapple, to make a smooth fairly runny batter. Pour batter into hot no-stick pan and place pineapple pieces evenly on batter. Put on lid and cook until firm. Serve with maple syrup

Almond Milk

3 tbsps almond meal
1 tspn vanilla essence
sprinkle cinnamon powder

1 tbsp honey
2 cups water

Combine all ingredients together in a blender and drink immediately or refrigerate until cool.

Method 2
1 cup almonds, soaked for 12 hours
5 cups water
    Place soaked almonds and 1 cup of water in blender. Blend

at medium speed until smooth. Add remaining water and blend at high speed for 2 min. Strain and store liquid in a glass jar in fridge for up to 4 days.

Rejuvalac

1 cup grain or seeds to sprout
fresh ginger to taste
large jar (1 lt)

Soak grain for 12 hours (summer) or 24 hours (winter). Drain off water and allow to sprout for 12-24 hours. Blend with 1 cup of water for 15 seconds and pour into jar, adding enough water to fill jar. Throw in the ginger and allow to sit at room temperature for 2 days then pour liquid through strainer. Keep the liquid in the fridge for several days.

Paneer Chenna

2 litres skim milk
3 to 6 tbsps fresh lemon juice

Paneer is fresh cheese made by souring hot milk with a little lemon juice and then pressing out the liquid until it becomes a firm mass.

The process is simple and quick. The soft cheese produced after the whey has drained is called *paneer chenna*. It is used in desserts, and it is an ingredient in a number of savoury dishes. When paneer chenna is pressed under a heavy weight for an hour or two, it firms up and becomes *paneer tikki*, or wedge cheese, used commonly in north Indian dishes.

Paneer tikki has little taste of its own, but it has a delightful texture. Unlike most cheeses, it keeps its firmness even when heated, rather than melting. You will need a colander, cheesecloth, a deep heavy, non-reactive saucepan, a wooden spoon, a large bowl, and a heavy weight. Place a colander lined with three or four layers of cheesecloth over a large bowl.

In a heavy non-reactive saucepan, heat the milk gradually to boiling, stirring occasionally with a wooden spoon to keep it from scorching or from forming a skin. Then lower the heat to medium and add lemon juice 1 tablespoon at a time, stirring gently with a wooden spoon for 15 to 20 seconds after you add each tablespoon. The milk may turn with as little as 2 tablespoons lemon juice, but it may take more, so be patient; when it turns, the whiter curds will separate from the pale green whey, so both the colour and texture of the milk will change.

As soon as the milk starts to turn, remove it from the heat. Stir for another few seconds, and then pour into the cloth-lined colander.

Rinse briefly under slow-running cold water to remove the lemon taste. Gather the edges of the cheesecloth together, squeeze out the water, then knot together the cheesecloth (or loop a rubber band around it) to create a bag you can hang from a hook. Rinse out the bowl and place under the cheesecloth bag to catch the drips of whey.

After only 20 min. you will have a soft cheese, paneer chenna. To make paneer tikki take the bag down, but don't untie it, and flatten the lump of chenna into an approximately 10 cm. square. Leaving it covered with the cheesecloth, place it on a plate or on a counter top and flatten it with a heavy weight to compress it into the dense-textured cheese. Press the cheese for 2 hours. Remove from the cheesecloth and use immediately, or store in plastic wrap in the refrigerator.

Seed Cheese

1 cup rejuvalac
2 cups sunflower or sesame seeds (soaked for 8 hours)

Pour the rejuvalac into a blender, blend at high speeds and slowly add the seeds until smooth. Pour into a glass jar or dish and set aside for 4-8 hours to ferment. Pour off the whey and place in an airtight container. This will keep for about 5 days in the fridge.

Seed Dressing

½ eschallot finely chopped
½ cucumber finely chopped
½ red capsicum finely chopped

1 cup seed cheese
1 tbsp tamari

Place all ingredients in a blender and blend at high speed for a couple of min. until smooth.

Root Ginger Drink

1 lt cold pure water
3 tbsps fresh grated ginger
½ lemon, sliced paper thin

2 tbsps honey (melted)
2 tbsps fresh lemon juice

Blend all ingredients, except lemon slices, in a blender. Serve chilled in tall glasses. Add crushed ice if desired. In each glass put 1 or 2 of the lemon slices.

CLEANSING JUICES

Juices are a great break for the digestive system as the juicer does most of the breaking down of the food and you are left with the good bits.

They should be drunk as they are made as many of the enzymes and vitamins. oxidise, or deactivate if exposed to air. They are best used as an adjunct to food that your body can digest and therefore use to repair and build. Any prolonged juice cleanses should only be done when resting and not in a working environment.

The energy from the juices should be available to do the cleansing and not cope with a hectic routine.

Juice cleansing is a way which gives the deepest, quickest cleansing and will help change habits and attitudes much more easily.

These are some of the juices we have found to be useful.

Apple and Lime

6 yellow and or red apples
¼ lime with rind on

This juice helps to cut through acidic wastes, clear stomach and bowels to assist in releasing old, stuck wind (don't have before big date!). Helps overworked kidneys as well.

Elixir Broth

2 medium carrots
½ medium parsnip
50 g mushrooms

4 egg tomatoes
2 sticks celery
4 brussel sprouts

¼ onion

3 cloves garlic

100 g green beans

2 yellow squash

½ zucchini

¼ cup mixed herbs

1 cm. cube ginger

This yummy vegetable juice alkalises and revitalises the entire system. It also helps the lungs and oxygenation. It may be taken as a cold juice at room temperature.

Heating deactivates some of the enzymes but the juice still retains the minerals and helps to heat the system.

Pear and Strawberry

6 Packenham pears

6-12 strawberries

Soothes the gall bladder and assists in the elimination of undigested fatty acids.

Grape and Lemon

¼ small lemon with rind on

500 g black grapes

Decongests, revitalises, cuts fatty acids, neutralises toxic matter and helps the spleen and gall bladder. Black grape remedies have been hailed as miracle cures for everything and there are many books written on grape remedies using juices and whole grapes. The best way is to avoid getting to that dire stage but for that small helping hand this is a great tonic.

APPENDIX

Tomatoes
To skin the tomatoes place into boiling water until the skin starts to blister. Remove from the water and peel away the skin and puree using either a blender or a potato masher.

Vegie salt
Salt flavoured with dried herbs and spices. Some are very 'salty' due to the amount of celery in the mixture which has a high amount of sodium of its own. Also ensure the salt is rock or Celtic salt and that there are no fillers.

Baking powder
To make your own use 1 part bicarbonate soda to 2 parts cream of tartar. Most brands have fillers or some sort of starch which make them unsuitable to combine with the flour (starch).

Setting point of jam
Place a spoonful onto a saucer or plate and put it into the freezer. Allow to stand for 5 min., then remove the plate and check consistency of the mixture. It should be fairly stiff and the surface wrinkled when ready for bottling. If not, return and reheat for a few more minutes. If using honey, the jam will usually turn out a little bit less set than by using sugar.

Sterilising jars

Wash thoroughly in hot soapy water, then rinse well in hot water. Place bottles on clean oven racks and heat to 150°C. Leave for about 5 min. and allow jars to cool slightly before using. Use jars with metal lids only.

Bread crumbs

The type you buy in the shops are going to have all the problems associated with the digestion of bread. Either use crumbs from bread you have made yourself or bought bread, which has one type of flour and water only, i.e., no yeast, sugar, etc.

If you want to mix the crumbs with proteins, starches or fatty acids then you will need to use crumbs from sprouted bread. To use dry the bread slowly in oven or pan until you are able to crumble it. Dry longer if necessary after you have crumbed it.

Vanilla Essence

1 vanilla bean
2 tbsps honey
250 ml water

Roughly chop the vanilla bean and place in saucepan with the other ingredients. Bring slowly to the boil then simmer for about 10 min. Strain and save the liquid and store in bottle in fridge.

Lemon Grass Tea

To make lemon grass tea you may use either fresh or dried lemon grass. If this is not available, a tea bag will do. The strength of the tea will vary with the freshness of the lemon grass, but as a rule half a cup of lemon grass steeped in 2 cups of boiling water will make a decent strength stock. As always adjust the amount to suit your tastes.